This book belongs to:

Rachel

Steinhart

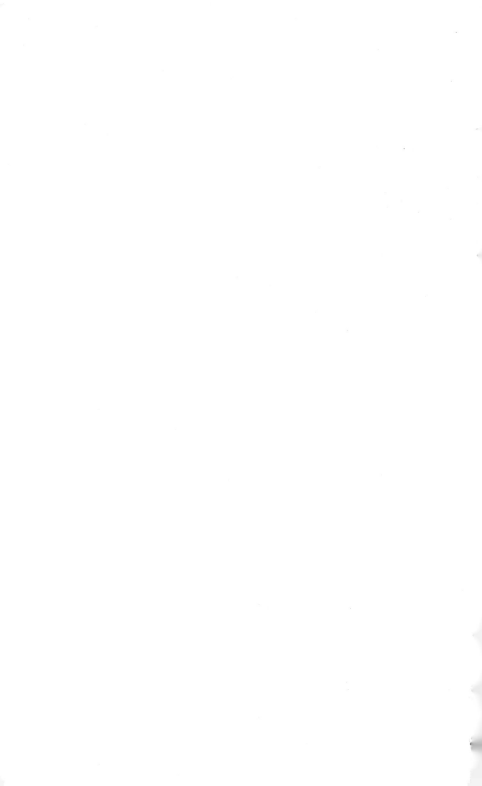

THE
DOCTOR–ACTIVIST

Physicians Fighting for
Social Change

THE DOCTOR–ACTIVIST
Physicians Fighting for Social Change

Edited by
ELLEN L. BASSUK

Better Homes Fund
and Harvard Medical School
Newton Center, Massachusetts

With the assistance of
REBECCA W. CARMAN

PLENUM PRESS • NEW YORK AND LONDON

Library of Congress Cataloging-in-Publication Data

On file

ISBN 0-306-45267-7

© 1996 Plenum Press, New York
A Division of Plenum Publishing Corporation
233 Spring Street, New York, N.Y. 10013-1578

10 9 8 7 6 5 4 3 2 1

To *Fella Cederbaum*. With gratitude and love for guiding me along the path to truth and freedom: The eagle will soar.

FOREWORD

This is a timely book for all interested in social progress. These autobiographical accounts of physicians' struggles to improve the lives of people need to be told, for we live in a time when there is considerable skepticism about the role of physicians in creating social change.

Let me explain. In the United States the delivery of health services — especially the financing of these services — has been transformed. The management of much of medical care has been moved into large-scale for-profit corporate entities. The nonprofit sector, defensively, has begun to behave like the for-profit sector. This has resulted in what has been referred to as the "corporatization" of medicine and the "proletarianization" of the medical profession. Will this leave room for the kind of social activism by physicians recorded in this volume?

The organized medical profession in the United States unfortunately has not provided congenial auspices for physicians as social activists. Justifiably or not, these organizations are publicly perceived as being preoccupied with their self-interests rather than with the public's health. This caused one president of the American Academy of Pediatrics to state in his presidential address that "when pediatricians talk about what is good for the pediatricians, no one will listen. When they talk about what is good for the children, everyone will listen."

But social activist physicians have been inventive. They have developed new organizations as outlets for their concerns about the health and welfare of people around the world. Thus, among many others, Physicians for Social Responsibility, Physicians for Human Rights, and the International Physicians for the Prevention of Nuclear War have become significant social forces. The last organization's contributions were recognized with the award of the Nobel Peace Prize. These organizations figure prominently in the lives of this generation of doctor–activists.

As one reads of the lives of these physicians, the eclectic nature of their activities is impressive. Certainly there is no cookie cutter from which they have been stamped. Yet while their activities have been very diverse, there does seem to be a core of attributes which, in my view, they share. Among these are:

1. A clear social conscience, by which I mean a deeply held commitment to helping others. While we don't know all of the roots of social conscience (indeed the literature is sparse), we do hear from each of these authors about the importance of early experiences in shaping this commitment. The roots clearly antedate embarking on a career in medicine.

2. Inventiveness in the applications of their medical knowledge in developing new ways to bring more and better services to a larger number of people. Their rootedness in medical knowledge is part of what makes them unique.

3. Courage. All of these authors were self-propelled to the point of pursuing their goals in the face of opposition and/or criticism that often caused them to be labeled impractical, or dreamers, or worse. They persevered when they were told, "it can't be done."
4. A high energy level. Clearly these activists had to function with extraordinary expenditures of energy to accomplish their goals.
5. Resourcefulness. All manifested innovative ways of bringing people and programs together in more effective arrangements.

All of these attributes add up to creativity. Each of these people knew when to seize the initiative to implement their programs. Several authors indicate specifically that they could not plan to do what they ultimately accomplished, but they recognized when a somewhat fortuitous set of circumstances made it possible for them to act. They are examples of what Louis Pasteur recognized when he said, "chance favors the prepared mind."

In the Overview the editor properly points to the rich history of social activism by physicians. Among these activists is Dr. William Henry Welch, the first dean of the Johns Hopkins School of Medicine, who played an important role in bringing together medical education, research, and service into the four-year curriculum that has come to be recognized as modern medical education. He recognized that the advances in the natural sciences had to be incorporated into medical education and that preceptorial teaching was no longer sufficient. In the process the teaching hospital and its outpatient services became an integral part of educating physicians.

Another of Dr. Welch's contributions relates to his keen sense of history. In 1891 he arranged to honor the 70th birthday of a person who may be the model doctor–activist of all time, Dr. Rudolf Virchow. At that time Welch said,

To appreciate the character and extent of an advance made by scientific discovery, it is necessary to know something about the ideas which have been displaced or overthrown by the discovery. The younger generation of students are in danger of forgetting that facts which are taught to them and which seem to them the simplest and the most natural, may have cost years of patient investigation and hard controversy, and possibly have taken the place of doctrines, very different or even contradictory, which long held sway, and which seemed to other generations equally simple and natural.

Virchow is regarded as the founder of cellular pathology and as an important contributor to the establishment of scientific medicine. He carried on his scholarly activities in pathology while becoming an activist to promote the democratic revolutions sweeping across Europe in his time. He wrote,

The democratic state desires that all its citizens enjoy a state of well-being, for it recognizes that they all have equal rights . . . it is not enough for the state to guarantee every citizen the basic necessities for existence, and to assist everyone whose labor does not suffice for him to acquire these necessities; the state must do more, it must assist everyone so far that he will have the conditions necessary for a healthy existence.

Dr. Virchow served on commissions to investigate epidemics and in the process virtually invented modern public health. He campaigned for compulsory meat inspection as a consequence of his studies of trichinosis. At the request of the Berlin City Council he designed and supervised a sewage disposal system which was widely copied. Most of all he saw the relationship between health and social conditions and wrote of medicine as a social science. He thought of physicians as the natural attorneys for the poor and believed that social problems fall within their jurisdiction.

Dr. Welch's commitment to scholarship in medical history led him to lay the groundwork for an Institute on the History of Medicine at Johns Hopkins. The university had the wisdom to recruit the great physician–medical historian, Dr. Henry Sigerist from Europe. This not only brought professionalism to the study of medical history, but it brought Dr. Sigerist's social vision of medicine's responsibility to society to the university. Indeed, prior to World War II, Dr. Sigerist and his historian colleague, George Rosen at Yale, not only wrote extensively about the history of what they called social medicine, but in addition were themselves social activists. They advocated studies of programs for national health insurance and encouraged cross-national studies of medical care systems. Medical students across the country were greatly influenced by their teachings and writings. It is fair to say that many of the physician–activists of the last several decades were stimulated by these scholars. I am sure I would do some injustice if I attempted to list them all. Several of them are mentioned as mentors in these accounts.

In reading these autobiographical accounts, one is impressed by many insights. On a personal note, as an activist I can't help but resonate to the conclusion of Dr. Jack Geiger's chapter. He indicates the generic issue is, "Watch for the moment — the opportunity — that reflects your values. Seize it."

It brought back memories of 1965 when, as professor of pediatrics at the State University of New York at Syracuse, I was carrying on research with Dr. Bettye Caldwell on the development of young children growing up in poverty. We documented their decline in development; but more important, we also showed that we could prevent the decline with enrollment of the children in a comprehensive child care program in the preschool years.

The "moment" came. As we were making our observations, President Johnson and the Congress established the Office of Economic Opportunity. The first Director, Mr. Sargent Shriver, had heard of our work and wanted to know if we could replicate our work on a national scale. Without the clinical experience and demonstration we had made, I might have been hesitant. But it was clear that the time would not come again. So with the help of many talented people, we created the Head Start Program. Within 6 months we mounted a comprehensive child development summer program for 500,000 preschool children in 2700 communities across the nation. It is now a year-round program. Unfortunately it has not grown to reach all of the eligible children, since only about one-third of them are enrolled.

Since I was the only physician in the Office of Economic Opportunity, I soon became the assistant to the director for health affairs. I recalled the report of a remarkable group, the Committee on the Cost of Medical Care, which I had read as a medical student in 1935. Among many other significant recommendations (most of which were never acted upon because we were then in the midst of the Great Depression) it proposed the establishment of community health centers to provide medical care for the unserved and underserved groups. At the time we were thinking of how to implement such a program, we received the proposal from Drs. Count Gibson and Jack Geiger (building on his experience in South Africa) to establish two centers, one in urban Boston and one in rural Mound Bayou, Mississippi — as is so well described in Dr. Geiger's chapter. We went on in those early days to fund 50 centers; ultimately this network grew to more than 800 community health centers after the program was transferred to the Department of Health, Education, and Welfare.

I return to the fact that the editor has done us a service by collecting these interesting autobiographical accounts of doctor–activists. I can't help, however, calling attention to the many less visible activists who have provided health services in so many ways for those in need. I think of the many Peace Corps physicians whose lives were enriched through service; the many physicians serving in nongovernmental organizations in the field of international health who have worked so hard to bring better health to people all over the world; and the many who organized rural and urban health clinics and clinics for migrant workers, Native Americans—and many others in addition to those recorded in this volume. They all "watched for the moment . . ." and "seized it."

An overarching challenge remains. The subtitle of this book is "Physicians Fighting for Social Change." Can the collective wisdom and experience lead the many physician–activists to develop social strategies that will provide all of the people of the world with appropriate health care? This is the goal enunciated by the Director General of the World Health Organization, Dr. Halfden Mahler, when he declared at the World Health Assembly in 1978: "Health for all by the year 2000." Clearly much work remains to be done.

JULIUS B. RICHMOND, M.D.
Professor of Health Policy, Emeritus
Department of Social Medicine
Harvard Medical School

PREFACE

In writing a preface to a book of autobiographies, it seems natural to throw in a good measure of self-reflection, revisiting a vast array of formative childhood experiences and important life junctures. I have resisted this temptation, instead focusing on the circumstances that drew me toward this project. I believe that the primary reason I chose to design and edit this volume lies in my personal commitment to a life of social activism and, in particular, my ongoing astonishment and outrage at the social injustices complicating the lives of extremely poor people, especially those who have special needs.

I often muse about how I wandered from my chosen profession of clinical psychiatry to serving as president of the Better Homes Fund, an organization that supports homeless families and children. The simple explanation — I said "yes" to a phone query — sheds little light on the factors in my background preparing me for this position or the unique opportunities I felt this new role would provide. Severe poverty and homelessness were not new to me; for more than a decade I have worked full-time in this area.

However, before assuming leadership at the Better Homes Fund I sometimes felt frustrated by my inability to help my patients improve their lives. I needed a vantage point from which to see and affect the interaction among individual vulnerabilities, socioeconomic circumstances, and policy and programmatic interventions.

More than a decade ago I was practicing psychiatry in a community-oriented teaching hospital in an urban setting, caring for people with severe mental illness. In the early days of my career I was a practitioner, clinically involved with people who had suffered inordinately, were challenged daily because of their differences, and often led desperately lonely lives. Through my work running an aftercare clinic and supervising residents on a psychiatric emergency ward, I sat face to face with despair. In the early 1980s, I saw troubled individuals confronted with new and even harsher realities — the low-income housing crisis, cutbacks in benefits to the poor, and the bleak aftermath of desinstitutionalization. More and more, our attempts to help people were stymied by inadequate resources and enormous gaps in available services. Now many people with chronic mental illness were faced not only with their internal experience and the stigma associated with it but also with the crippling burden of surviving without shelter. What was already a challenging job became virtually impossible as the single-room-occupancy residences were razed and housing became even more scarce. My only alternative was to constantly improvise, attempting to create referral options where none really existed. As my own anxiety and guilt mounted, I decided to quit my job and figure out some alternative way to respond to the enormity of these problems.

Not long afterwards I was asked to chair a community task force on homelessness. I visited a shelter and, to my surprise, it seemed similar to the back wards of the state

mental hospital where I had been a resident. My naive reaction was to try to educate policy makers about the great
numbers of people suffering from mental illness. I fully expected that if they understood the scope of the problem, they
would respond. I also believed that research findings speak
volumes, so I mobilized some of my colleagues to join me in
collecting clinical information about the residents of one of
the model state shelters. In one of the first reports of its kind
in the country, we documented that the majority of shelter
guests suffered from chronic mental illness. People were unwilling to hear our full message, however, and accused us of
blaming the victim. This took place in the early 1980s, when
it was close to heresy to say that any homeless person suffered from mental illness. Before I knew it, I was immersed
in a political quagmire.

As time passed, my role as a practitioner and clinical
researcher in the homelessness area also seemed limited in
scope and disconnected from my real purpose. Clinical work,
although always rewarding, involved only small numbers of
people, and the problems of poverty — especially when cou-
pled with personal vulnerability — were systemic, dwarfing
the individual. How could I effectively care for someone when
obstacles to living a decent life were out of our control and
seemingly insurmountable? Research seemed to have the potential to address some of my concerns, but only if I could
translate my findings into social action. To this end, I completed some of the early studies about homeless children in
the mid-1980s and advocated for services to meet their needs.
Through this work I had the experience of using research
findings to advance action agendas, but it all seemed seren-
dipitous and indirect. And why spend precious resources of
money and time unless improvements become palpably evident in the lives of poor people? My career path had brought
me to a position where I could wrestle with issues of homelessness just as the numbers of women and children on the
streets began to skyrocket. But attacking poverty in the lives

of vulnerable individuals seemed to require more comprehensive and complex strategies than either clinical care or research alone could accomplish.

At this point, in 1987, I was presented with an unusual opportunity. David Jordan, then Editor-in-Chief of *Better Homes and Gardens* magazine, wanted to establish an organization that could help homeless mothers and children. I seized on the chance to take our research and evaluation findings and translate them into programs to help extremely poor families and children. Although ours was an unlikely marriage of interests, common values prevailed, and we set up the Better Homes Fund in 1988. I became president of the Fund — now a thriving nonprofit organization — and, with David's unflagging support, enacted a life-long dream to make some small difference in bettering the lives of others.

Over the last 7 years I have struggled to establish an organization healthy enough to support our admittedly ambitious mission. As the Fund gradually reached solid footing, I have had time to reflect about where I have traveled and to what purpose. The Fund has become a national clearinghouse for information about homelessness and extreme poverty and has attempted to bring our research, academic, and clinical experiences to help design and implement creative programs and policies. This journey has challenged me daily to understand who I am both personally and professionally. Working with extreme poverty and the despair and heartache surrounding it and understanding the personal tragedy and web of oppression that contribute to it are humbling indeed. I have had to face my original frustrations again and again and repeatedly try to answer the question of how we can be more effective in responding to what we are seeing. Some of my early heady idealism has been transformed into what I believe is a more realistic approach: each of us must do our part, however small, to try to make this world a better place to live in. My goals are more modest, but I think more realistic. On days that I spend many hours raising money or am blocked in attempts to help the neediest and most troubled among the homeless, I have to remind myself again of why I am doing this. Our work at the Better Homes Fund echoes some of the journeys of the doctors in this book; their passion, in turn, gives me more energy to continue. It is exciting and heartening to be a part of this volume.

How did this volume come about? As part of my interest in social issues, I work as an editor of a book series on social psychiatry for Plenum Press. This involves a constant search for new book ideas and authors with Mariclaire Cloutier, a senior editor at Plenum Press. A few years ago, she expressed an interest in autobiographical accounts, and we came up with the idea for a volume about doctor–activists. Although I was and remain much too busy, I felt that it was important to undertake this venture, especially because doctors nowadays are so commonly under siege. Medicine has a long history of social activism; I felt that the life stories of similarly committed contemporary doctors might broaden the popular view of medicine and serve as an inspiration to younger physicians struggling with their careers. From the very beginning, I have felt a deep commitment to this book's overarching purpose. And similarly, I feel tremendous admiration for the traits of humanity, social justice, and common ingenuity represented by these authors.

This book consists of ten chapters, most of which are autobiographical accounts written by selected physicians. Each chapter provides a first-hand account of the person's career path. I want to thank all of the physicians who agreed to tell their stories as well as my brother-in-law, Jeffrey Koplan, a physician who is now Executive Vice President and Director of the Prudential Center for Health Care Research in Atlanta, who helped write the overview and identify some of the authors. They are all remarkably busy people, and I appreciate their willingness to reflect on their experience and to write about it. Their contributions have been invaluable—to my mind resulting in an exciting, inspiring, and richly detailed collection of chapters.

I also want to thank each physician for agreeing to contribute royalties to a social cause. The monies from the sale of this book will be contributed to Kidstart, a program for homeless 3- to 5-year-olds that is currently located in 17 sites nationwide. The Better Homes Fund piloted Kidstart in 1990 as a unique response to the multiple needs of homeless preschoolers. Homeless families and children now constitute almost 43% of the homeless population, and the plight of young children who are spending critical developmental years on the streets is especially desperate. Kidstart programs help many of these youngsters before they enter the school setting, especially those with serious developmental delays. We are grateful to the authors for their willingness to contribute to this program.

Various other people made this book possible. Without the advice of T. Stephen Jones, Henry Kahn, and Joseph Keogh, I might not have found such a colorful group of physicians. Rebecca Carman has helped to edit this volume. She has worked tirelessly, made many, many phone calls to errant authors, and tolerated frequent scheduling changes. Her editorial comments have made this volume easier to read, and her contribution to writing the postscripts has been critical. Jayne Samuda has helped with the production of the manuscript — as always, with good humor.

I am extremely grateful to Mariclaire Cloutier at Plenum for giving me the opportunity to understand some of my own activities within the perspective of other physicians' lives. And finally, I would like to thank my own children, Danny and Sarah, and the many homeless children I have worked with for considerably enriching my life.

CONTENTS

CHAPTER I

PHYSICIANS FIGHTING FOR SOCIAL CHANGE

An Overview

ELLEN L. BASSUK, M.D., and
JEFFREY P. KOPLAN, M.D.

Today's often cynical views of medicine have rendered many of its founding goals and ideals barely recognizable. Over the past few decades, medicine's "persona" has evolved from a humanitarian endeavor to a high-tech, impersonal, money-making venture. For example, managed care is threatening to turn medicine primarily into a business, preventive strategies have been eclipsed by spectacular rescues and miraculous cures, and the schism in quality of care available for those who can and can't afford treatment has widened. Changes in medicine's fundamental identity have made it easy to lose sight of the principles that in previous eras not only influenced medicine but defined it.

During the era of modern medicine, some physicians have been consistently involved with social issues — a portion of these have functioned as social activists as well. Similar to their forebears, they have seen medicine in a larger social context and as a potential agent of social change. For example, in the Roman Empire, physicians dealt with environmental issues such as draining malarious swamps; in 19th-century England, doctors understood that the cholera epidemics were related to filth and initiated a broad set of sanitary reforms; and in the mid-1960s, physicians provided medical support to civil rights activists in Mississippi through the Medical Committee for Human Rights. However, like the mercurial fortunes of a political party, medical activism comes into favor and flourishes for various intervals and recedes into isolated pockets during others.

The physician's role over the centuries has retained one common denominator: doctors care for others. Although the 1990s have their share of socially active physicians, it is the unusual doctor who translates his or her caring into serving disenfranchised persons and into pathways for social change. More exceptional still is the physician whose concerns transcend individual patients and communities and instead focus on global issues affecting the future of our planet and even the human race. In light of the diversity of persons practicing medicine, it is not surprising that some have approached it as a business, some as a profession, some as a calling, and others as a means of addressing broader societal problems. The efforts of this latter group are the subject of this volume.

In this book, ten exceptional physicians describe the course of their careers. Many struggles have been advanced through their efforts, including civil rights, women's rights, peace, environmental protection, universal access to health care, and public health. Some physicians have emigrated to less developed areas, for example, providing health care on Native American reservations or in Third-World countries. Others have spent their lives providing medical care to disadvantaged, underserved patients, such as in inner-city clinics. These physicians are part of a large cadre of professionals who quietly toil in the trenches, fighting the daily battles necessary to provide quality care to disenfranchised people. Still others have directed their efforts toward various medical areas that are greatly influenced by social and environmental factors, such the struggles against malnutrition, AIDS, tobacco, and nuclear war. And still others have explored the frontiers of our consciousness. These physicians have ingeniously crafted careers for the betterment of those who are disenfranchised and ultimately for all of us. As a group, they share a desire to use the power of their skills and knowledge and the prestige of their profession to make a difference in the lives of others.

The doctors in this book are not meant to represent all socially concerned or "activist" physicians, nor do their areas of interest represent all relevant social areas. We selected them through the recommendations of others and the author's familiarity with their work. Certainly, many dozens of other health professionals have similar stories that would be at home in a volume such as this. However, the physicians' lives and careers discussed in this volume offer examples of values, choices, and behaviors that expand our perception of "medical practice" and provide models of potential pathways for people entering medicine. Collectively, these accounts provide insight into the hearts and minds of doctors interested in social context and fighting for social change and testimony to the critical role they play within their profession. Most important, the chapters that follow convey something of the remarkable spirit fueling their aspirations and commitments.

These physicians have led complex, exciting, and meaningful lives guided by their beliefs. They have manifested unwavering dedication motivated by deeply held values and accompanied by the prolonged expenditure of intense energy. Their autobiographic accounts are thus highly illuminating to those in the process of shaping their lives around community service. Considered together, their stories raise many of the salient issues confronting doctors who choose, create, and live an activist life. Each physician can indeed be a role model for those engaged in similar activities within a particular medical field, but the relevance of their lives ripples far beyond any circumscribed specialty or social arena.

COMPOSING A CAREER

The doctors in this volume have forged unusual career paths. Rather than retracing the well-established routes of traditional medicine — becoming a practitioner or academic researcher — these physicians have cobbled together unique combinations of activities. Often, these activities have brought them to unusual settings in this country and abroad and have led to other similarly unusual experiences. Unlike the conventional medical practitioner or academic, these physicians have in common a willingness to take life-changing risks and to enter unexplored professional territory.

Their professional identities are characterized by traits of adaptability and versatility. By redefining traditional roles, many have found ways of providing quality care in resource-scarce settings. Physicians working in the larger social arena display similar qualities that allow them to develop innovative solutions to both individual and community problems. Within each setting, their respective political, social, and medical concerns overlap and merge, guided by a constellation of values that are often unstated.

The doctors in this volume describe their deep commitment to multiple and often shifting causes. To the casual eye, these changes often occur without an obvious pattern. Deeply held beliefs and values seem to be the common threads in their careers. Although these physicians generally have not discussed their values explicitly in the chapters, their behavior reflects strong and passionate beliefs that they successfully translate into action and, sometimes, activism.

What seems to unify and guide the stories told by the physicians in this volume is this personal, often unstated, vision. John Mack, for example, recalls in his chapter his often negative views of experiences as he was living them. He felt at times that his life lacked unity and clear direction, and the decisions he made at various junctures seemed random, even chaotic. Donald Francis too claims he "had no plan." Mack further reflects on the process of retelling his story and concludes that, inevitably, a narrative emerges from which meaning can be derived. A powerfully held belief system creates the underpinning for Mack's and Francis's life story.

WHY SOCIAL ACTION? CHARACTER AND IDENTITY

Not every visionary is capable of implementing his or her ideas. Mary Catherine Bateson, in her book *Composing a Life*,[1] describes creative careers as "ongoing improvisations" requiring the continuous "discovery of new forms of flexibility" (p. 235). These physicians, particularly the practitioners, are able to see subtle connections within and between systems. They have the ingenuity to use a wide range of disparate tools to achieve their goals, quickly embracing new opportunities consistent with their values and stridently opposing circumstances that are out of line. To implement their vision, these physicians have little trouble crossing traditional disciplines and employing diverse perspectives.

As physicians' stories unfold, it becomes clear that at a certain point personal and professional risks become inconsequential in the pursuit of important goals. These doctors rarely mention the costs in terms of time or energy for relationships, family, leisure activities, and, in some instances, salaries. However, although they are filled with vigor for their chosen work, each contributor has limits that are hinted at in the respective chapters. For most, the balance is tipped toward work, with some significant personal sacrifices made at home. Their life work seems to unfold inexorably despite other pressures and demands.

None of the doctors recounts long hours of reflection about his or her chosen path. Their choices seem almost second nature, although sometimes the meaning of occupational twists and turns was not manifest at the time. In psychological terms, their choices were ego syntonic, that is, part of who they are, indicative of their core identity. Occasionally, physicians' choices took on added weight because of outright opposition or even threat, but in almost all cases their personal fortitude was overriding. Perhaps the agonizing commonly associated with making choices is largely absent because these physicians' routes simply mirror their inner worlds. When external and internal reality closely coincide, choices are a matter of course.

WHY SOCIAL ACTION? ROLE MODELS AND RELATIONSHIPS

Colby and Damon[2] studied persons they describe as "moral exemplars" — people who have demonstrated moral excellence in their lives. Not surprisingly, they found that this subgroup's career choices were not directly dictated by personal histories. Colby and Damon instead describe a complex and multilayered set of factors encompassing the influence of primary relationships and critical groups. Family history, formative experiences, and intellectual influences all indubitably affect career decisions. Collaborative relationships are especially noteworthy as transformative agents, maturing individuals so they can summon the courage to take on the next set of tasks.

Using Andrei Sakharov's life as one example, Colby and Damon describe how "transformative social influence continues through the life span. It is not contained alone in early experiences, in onetime dramatic incidents, or in determinative personality characteristics, although any of these may play a role. The chief operative force is social communication and support" (p. 15). They described the following paradox: how independently minded "moral exemplars" were guided by others, open to support and feedback, and able to learn from these relationships, which then became mutually energizing.

Most of the doctors in this volume describe important relationships with mentors and life-long colleagues who understood and supported their choices. In early manuscript drafts, long lists of inspiring groups and individuals were included; as editor, it was difficult to keep this list modest. Some of the doctors describe how, during difficult career transitions, they turned to mentors who supported their risk taking. Occasionally, they were disappointed, but for the most part these relationships acted as catalysts, allowing them to meet the next challenge headlong.

What led these physicians to make such unusual and enduring choices? It would be facile to attribute physicians' choices to single determinants, and when we consider determinants together some mystery still remains. Explanations seem inadequate. An ineffable quality helps each person improvise and persist along extremely challenging career paths.

COMMON VALUES AND BELIEF SYSTEMS

Like many physicians, the doctors in this volume are committed to improving the well-being of their patients both as individuals and collectively. As a group, these physicians tend to be particularly interested in prevention and early intervention. Many come from public health backgrounds in which the health of the community is the primary focus.

Many of these physicians are also concerned about the environments people are born into and grow up in and how they contribute to or detract from wellness. Focus on this issue alongside an emphasis on treatment principles such as prevention is consistent with a larger vision — to increase the prospects of disadvantaged people and to improve their health and well-being. In short, they are interested in positively affecting multiple aspects of a patient's life. The variety of physicians' activities is subsumed by their common dedication to reducing suffering; this goal, underscored throughout this volume, both focuses and provides momentum to their lives.

Each of the doctors in this volume seems to share an ethos of caring and concern for patients, community, and even humankind. But as the chapters demonstrate, none of these physicians can be described as a naive do-gooder with good intentions but little real impact. Their resoluteness of purpose and, in some instances, their moral courage have been translated into actions that were effective in reaching their goals.

These physicians' career paths reflect a deep respect for others, including those who are very different. This value goes hand in hand with a belief in the interconnectedness of people, most evident in their capacity for empathy and compassion and their willingness to care for patients from diverse cultures and in faraway lands. Many traditional physicians only reluctantly care for people who are different, whether on the basis of ethnicity, poverty, or individual characteristics (e.g., mental illness, sexual preference). However, the doctors in this volume seem to relish diversity in patient care. For them, the prospects of disadvantaged people seem inextricably tied to their own and their children's futures. They use caretaking opportunities to learn and to grow and emerge from the experience much richer.

Overall, the activities of the doctors in this book reflect a larger ethos: concern about context and collective experience, whether in the culture, community, cosmos, or even beyond. By dedicating their energies to making the world a better place in which to live, these physicians seem to operate on a bigger scale and in larger arenas than many of their counterparts. And their path is punctuated by compassion, intense energy, and commitment to moral issues — a stance that benefits us all.

DISCUSSION

As exemplars of their profession and role models for future generations of physicians, the life stories of the doctors in this volume are instructive. Certainly their life stories help to embellish the medical profession and reduce some of the cynicism about doctors as mere technologists or businessmen, but their commitments and activities impact us all. They have a ripple effect in our society, suggesting how individual acts of dedication and compassion can help to make the world a better place. One can only hope their stories will inspire more of us to make commitments affecting our brethren, remembering that ultimately we are all interdependent.

As the Tibetan Buddhist master Soygal Rinpoche observed[3]:

> Think of a tree. When you think of a tree, you tend to think of a distinctly defined object; and on a certain level, like the wave it is. But when you look more closely at the tree, you will see that ultimately it has no independent existence. When you contemplate it, you will find that it dissolves into an extremely subtle net of relationships that stretches across the universe. The rain that falls on its leaves, the wind that sways it, the soil that nourishes and sustains it, all the seasons and the weather, moonlight and starlight and sunlight — all form part of the tree. As you begin to think about the tree more and more, you will discover that everything in the universe helps to make the tree what it is; that it cannot at any moment be isolated from anything else; and that at every moment its nature is subtly changing (pp. 37–38).

In the subsequent pages, ten physicians tell their stories of social commitment. Consistent with the time-honored tradition of social action in medicine, these doctors have committed their lives to helping others by attending to social context. Just like the tree, their activities have been fostered by many complex factors and relationships and in turn have impacted profoundly on the people and communities they have served. They have made the world a better place to live in and are role models for all of us.

REFERENCES

1. Bateson MC: *Composing a Life*. New York: Penguin Books, 1989.
2. Colby A, Damon W: *Some Do Care. Contemporary Lives of Moral Commitment*. New York: The Free Press, 1992.
3. Rinpoche S: *The Tibetan Book of Living and Dying*. San Francisco: Harper San Francisco, 1992.

SUGGESTED READING

Horn J: *Away with All Pests. An English Surgeon in People's China: 1954–1969*. New York: Monthly Review Press, 1969.

Morantz-Sanchez RM: *Sympathy and Science. Women Physicians in American Medicine*. New York: Oxford University Press, 1985.

McNeill W: *Plagues and Peoples*. New York: Anchor Books, 1976.

Sidel V, Sidel R (eds): *Reforming Medicine: Lessons of the Last Quarter Century*. New York: Pantheon Books, 1984.

Verghere A: *My Own Country. A Doctor's Story of a Town and Its People in the Age of AIDS*. New York: Simon & Schuster, 1994.

CHAPTER II

A LIFE IN SOCIAL MEDICINE

H. JACK GEIGER, M.D.

Any autobiographical task is full of traps and seductions, most particularly the temptation to describe one's career as linear and logical — the consequence of a series of carefully planned and rational choices. The truth is grittier than that. Most of us, I think, stumble into our futures. The ultimate importance of some choices is rarely clear at the time they are made, and critical junctures are often identifiable only in hindsight. Defining and living out an identity in medicine may indeed be driven by some central convictions, but this process is also a disorderly mixture of luck, of some opportunities seized and others missed, and of a few rare moments of inspiration.

These moments of inspiration, I believe, almost always consist of a synthesis of earlier experiences and values — a series of links extending at least as far back as adolescence — and the sudden realization of their relevance to the tasks that medicine faces.

11

One of those moments came early in my third year in medical school at Case–Western Reserve. From the upper floors of the school I could see past the teaching hospitals into the city of Cleveland. It occurred to me that, out there, who got sick and who did not, what happened to them next, and their interactions with the medical care system were all social as well as biological phenomena. And something further — some half-formed questions came to mind. If (as I had begun to realize) the social and biological and physical environments, not medical care, were the real determinants of the health of any population, why couldn't that equation be run backwards? Why couldn't medical care be used to intervene in those environments? Why not make medicine an instrument of social change?

Later, in the library, I discovered that Virchow and the British pioneers in social medicine had been asking such questions for almost a century. These questions were to lead me first to South Africa, later to places as disparate as rural Mississippi and inner-city Boston. Their pursuit informed the core of my work and ultimately led me to try to develop a new role for medicine in the tragedies in Kurdistan and Iraq, the West Bank and Gaza Strip, and the former Yugoslavia.

I came to medical school late — I was almost 30 — after devoting myself almost entirely to civil rights and writing. I finished high school in New York when I was 14, and no college would admit me at that age. Frustrated and adrift, I left my middle-class family, took a job as a copyboy at the *New York Times,* and found a new home with the family of an outstanding black actor, Canada Lee. Through that apartment — a penthouse atop Sugar Hill in Harlem — came the leaders of the African-American political and arts communities: Richard Wright, Langston Hughes, Adam Clayton Powell, Jr., Josh White, A. Philip Randolph, the young James Baldwin, and many others. All I had to do was listen; it would have been an extraordinary educational opportunity for anyone, but particularly for one who was white. A year later, at the University of Wisconsin, I worked at night as a journalist and campaigned against university-sanctioned racial and religious discrimination in housing. I also joined in founding the second chapter of the Congress of Racial Equality (CORE), a new civil rights organization. Adopting Gandhian techniques of direct confrontation and non-violent resistance, CORE fought to end discrimination in defense plants. In 1943, I enlisted in the U.S. Merchant Marine — the only service, in World War II, that was not racially segregated — and sailed for years on the only American vessel with an interracial officer crew and a black captain, Hugh Mulzac.

From 1947 to 1953, I studied science at the University of Chicago. During the next 4 years, I reported on the unfolding of a golden age in biological research, attending the scientific conferences, reading the papers, and interviewing the scientists. I could not fail to note the convergence of virology, genetics, and enzymology in research on the nucleic acids, and I was fascinated. A future Nobel laureate, Salvatore Luria, gave me the courage to be serious. During an interview on his work on lysogeny, I asked a question — a very good question, he said — and he offered me a job as a graduate student. In 1954, I decided instead to quit my job, go to medical school, and do research on DNA (an easier route to research, I thought, than a Ph.D.) And then, 3 years later, I came to the aforementioned questions and to my interest in social medicine.

Most of what passed for social or community medicine in the United States in those days, it seemed to me, was merely rhetorical — it wasn't something you did; it was an attitude you held. Then I came across an article describing what seemed to be a *real* program in, of all places, South Africa. The program was administered through the University of Natal, which was at that time the country's only medical school for nonwhites. Directed by the pioneering physician Sidney Kark, it consisted of a set of rural and urban community health centers serving Zulu populations. Somehow I stitched together 5 months of elective and vacation time, found funding for myself and my wife, obtained the necessary permissions, and flew to Africa. I was seizing the moment, and it was to change my life.

In 1940, Kark and his colleagues created the first modern comprehensive community health center at Polela, a 500-square-mile desperately poor rural area in a Zulu "tribal reserve." Over the next 5 years, they added five more health centers to serve African, Asian, and poor white urban communities, created an Institute of Family and Community Health in Durban, and, in 1954, incorporated the whole operation as the Department of Social Medicine at the University of Natal. Social medicine at the Institute emphasized practice in real communities as well as theory and a strategy of community diagnosis and intervention known later as community-oriented primary care.

I was put to work in the health center at Lamontville, an African housing project of 22,000 people on the edge of Durban. It was a clerkship, I think, unlike any other. Zulu community organizers walked me through the endless jumble of cinder-block homes and squatters' shacks and taught me the social structure of a community that mixed people from a half-dozen tribal origins and languages with second-generation urban residents and just-arrived rural migrants. Public health nurses took me on their rounds and indicated which subgroups were at special risk.

I also received a crash course in environmental sanitation. My first patient, a mother of seven, had typhoid fever, her oldest child had tuberculosis, and her youngest had severe malnutrition. On the wall of my examining room hung a long row of epidemiologic charts for Lamontville: rates of infant mortality and hypertension, incidence and prevalences of infectious disease, growth and weight curves by family composition and income, social networks, and charts of ethnic origins.

Later, in the health center serving the thatched huts and clustered hilltop villages of Polela, the same message came through. One never merely saw an individual patient; one saw patient, family, and community, with the community as the ultimate focus of concern. The disciplines of epidemiology, the social sciences, and biology were the basis for intervention in whole communities; this process was as central as clinical diagnoses and treatments of individuals.

When I returned to my senior year of medical school in Cleveland, I thought that my work would be in international health. I chose my training carefully to prepare for that role: internship and residencies in medicine on the Harvard service of Boston City Hospital, serving the poor; a fellowship in infectious disease, a public health degree in epidemiology, and postdoctoral studies in medical social sciences.

By then it was 1964, and I was planning to go to work in a health center in Nigeria. This was the year of the long, hot "Freedom Summer" in the South, with people registering voters and campaigning for civil rights, and many being beaten and killed in the struggle. I postponed the assignment to Africa and, with many others, helped to found the Medical Committee for Human Rights. Along with hundreds of other physicians, nurses, and health worker volunteers, I headed for Mississippi to help provide medical care, support, and protection for civil rights workers. I took a long, close look at the poverty, misery, and deprivation — and, inevitably, illness — in the sharecropper shacks and small-town black slums of the deep South. Gradually, it became clear that one didn't have to go to Africa, Southeast Asia, or Latin America to find poverty. There was a third world within the United States: blacks and Hispanics in the urban ghettos, blacks in the rural south, Mexican-Americans in the Southwest, poor whites in Appalachia, and Native Americans on reservations.

At a meeting of civil rights activists in Greenville, Mississippi, I described Polela and Lamontville and suggested the development of a community health center model in the United States with an American medical school taking the lead. The United States had had "health centers" before —

the term covered many different models — but they were, almost without exception, public health clinics, limited to well-baby and preventive services. (One such network mollified organized medicine with the motto "No diagnoses made, no prescriptions written.") Most importantly, these centers lacked any mandate for social and political action.

A fellow volunteer, Count Gibson, then chairman of preventive medicine at Tufts Medical School in Boston, offered his department. And we were lucky: there was a brand-new government agency, the Office of Economic Opportunity (OEO), proclaiming its commitment to social change as part of the "War on Poverty." We took the idea of a Polela-like health center to the OEO and made the familiar arguments. Why couldn't community health centers be used as a route to social, economic, and political change — addressing the deepest causes of disease? And shouldn't we have a new model for primary care that would draw on the resources of the people themselves, making them active rather than passive participants?

Six months later, OEO approved our first grant for two health centers — one at Columbia Point, a 6000-person urban housing project on the edge of downtown Boston, and the other in Mound Bayou, a town of 12,000 black rural people in northern Bolivar County, Mississippi. Then and now, this county, located in the heart of the Mississippi Delta, is one of the poorest areas in the nation. In effect, we had replicated Lamontville and Polela.

Both centers developed the essentials of community-oriented primary care: family health care teams; community organization and health education; the training of local workers as family health aides, environmental sanitarians, and health educators; and an emphasis on demography and epidemiology.

But there was a difference, most evident in the Delta. The Mound Bayou Health Council — the community governing board — was chartered as a community development corporation. This program included early child care, nutritional and social programs for the isolated rural elderly, a bus transportation system, legal services, and housing rehabilitation. Plans for a community vegetable garden grew into the 600-acre North Bolivar County Farm Cooperative. This farm, which grew vegetables instead of cotton, was owned by a thousand of the poorest families in the area, who traded their labor for shares in the food crop.

Most important was an in-service training program that grew into a full-fledged Office of Education, with high-school equivalency and college preparatory courses taught at night by health center professionals and assistance in making applications and finding scholarships. In the first decade alone, that program produced seven M.D.s, five Ph.D.s, more than 20 registered nurses and social workers, the first ten registered black sanitarians in Mississippi (two of whom went on to earn environmental engineering degrees), and a host of technicians. These successful participants reinforce an important lesson: the communities of the poor — places the public are taught to regard as sinkholes of pathology — are full of untapped human resources, people with drive and intelligence and the commitment to achieve if given half a chance.

The years in Mississippi were full of struggle and were among the happiest of my life. Black professionals, people born in Mississippi who had migrated north, returned to work at the health center: John Hatch, a social worker who became director of community organization and health education; Andrew James, an environmental expert who ran a massive well-digging, privy-building, house-rehabilitating program; and Dr. Helen Barnes, an obstetrician-gynecologist who directed family planning and nurse-midwifery programs. They worked alongside white recruits, mostly physicians and nurses, from the North. Local residents filled more and more of the health center jobs, used their salaries to build decent homes and send their children to college, and taught us all lessons about resilience in the face of adversity. I felt astonishment and exhilaration at what had been unleashed — that all this was happening. I can remember walking through the empty small-town streets of Mound Bayou late at night just to look at the health center, located in what had been a cotton field only a few years earlier, to assure myself that it was really there.

We spent time training the staffs of other health centers, for in a few years there were many. The original Tufts projects were followed by four others — in Chicago, the Bronx, Los Angeles, and Denver. Then, after Senator Ted Kennedy visited Columbia Point, Congress passed legislation authorizing a national network of community health centers. These grew during the 1970s to total more than 600 and were the primary sources of health care for nearly 7 million low-income, mostly minority Americans. Unique in the U.S. health care system, they are controlled by the people they serve. By law, each of the health center governing boards must have a majority of members who are users of the service.

But those years came at a cost. I was acting chairman of the Department of Community Medicine at Tufts, director of the Columbia Point Health Center, and director of the Delta Center, 1500 miles away. I had two homes, a trailer in Mound Bayou and an apartment in Boston. There was constant travel, in addition, to recruit staff, defend budgets, and speak to medical, public health, and civil rights groups. Bitter conflicts arose — first with the white power structure in Mississippi and then in a series of social class struggles within the black community, as control of budgets, jobs, and educational opportunities moved from an existing middle-class elite to the rural poor. The work was consuming, and my absences long; finally, the family pressures became intolerable and ended in divorce.

With the advent of the Nixon administration in 1968, OEO was undermined and began to deteriorate (all of the health centers were later transferred to the Department of Health, Education and Welfare). The Columbia Point Health

Center sought independence from Tufts — the right outcome for a program committed to community control. In its dying days, OEO transferred the Delta Health Center to a local group — but, in my view, to the wrong local group: not the Health Council, elected by the county's rural poor, but a Mound Bayou-based middle-class group associated with a small community hospital, also an OEO grantee. My work in Mississippi, I thought, was over. The health center was still there, but in both sociopolitical and personal terms, I believed I had lost.

It was a time of considerable despair. I had moved to the new medical school at the State University of New York at Stony Brook, on Long Island, but the school's promised focus on community medicine failed to materialize. Further, although I had been comfortable on inner-city streets and rural cotton fields, I now felt adrift in exurban slurb, a place where the center of community life seemed to be the shopping mall. In a 4-year period beginning in 1974, both of my parents suffered terminal cancers, and my former wife died of the sequelae of an automobile accident. I felt alone, depressed, and unproductive — failed.

Salvation — I use the word advisedly — began suddenly, with a new opportunity. City College, the Harlem campus of the City University of New York, began a pioneering medical school explicitly committed to the recruitment of underrepresented minorities and to training students specifically for primary care in the inner city. In 1978, the school created a chair in community medicine and offered me the position. I jumped at the chance to return to my adolescent roots, to blend civil rights and medicine, and to develop a curriculum in community-oriented primary care. Above all, I wanted to join in another effort to recognize and develop the strengths that exist in impoverished populations. I have been there ever since.

The City University of New York Medical School gave me and my departmental colleagues an extensive share of the curriculum and great flexibility. Our students receive 3 years of teaching and experience in community medicine — a program without parallel in conventional medical schools. Significant portions of these years are spent in community health centers and other health-related community-based organizations. Students learn to think about the health of populations, not just individual patients, and they acquire the epidemiologic, survey research, and evaluation tools to make community diagnoses and plan interventions.

For many people in academic community medicine, the usual medical school responsibilities of teaching and research comprise only one part of what they see as their work. Almost all of us are involved in extracurricular social and political action on health-related issues in the larger society. For me, the civil rights and health care of the poor had been the central concern.

And then, in 1980, a new crusade began. The election of Ronald Reagan brought with it a presidential conviction that nuclear war was "winnable," a massive expansion of the American nuclear arsenal, and the onset of a deadly and dangerous nuclear arms race. Almost two decades earlier, in 1961, I had been one of a group of young physicians convened by a dynamic and world-famous Boston cardiologist, Dr. Bernard Lown. We had gathered in shocked response to the administration's promise that nuclear war was survivable — all you had to do, they said, was build a little fallout shelter in your backyard. Our study group conducted a serious, independent scientific and medical examination of the consequences of a defined nuclear attack on the United States. The results, published in a special issue of the *New England Journal of Medicine* early in 1962, were terrifying. We found that even a modest attack (trivial by the standards of the 1990s) would be devastating, causing tens of millions of simultaneous deaths and destroyed institutions. Without precedent in human experience, an attack would irreparably rip the social fabric, making recovery impossible. The medical community, but not the politicians, paid attention.

The study group became an organization, Physicians for Social Responsibility (PSR), and turned its attention to the consequences of atmospheric testing of nuclear weapons, then the norm. We had an early triumph: demonstrating the presence of radioactive strontium-90 in the baby teeth of infants in St. Louis, a city in the middle of the fallout pathway. In less than a year, President Kennedy signed the Partial Nuclear Test Ban Treaty outlawing tests in the atmosphere.

But the Vietnam War was growing apace, and the convulsive national debate that followed swept away all other issues. By the early 1970s, PSR was dormant. Now, in 1980, it was time to renew it. A charismatic Boston pediatrician, Dr. Helen Caldicott, led the way; over the next few years, PSR's membership grew to more than 30,000 physicians and supporters, including most of the original founders.

The study of the medical, biological, and social consequences of nuclear war had to be done all over again, for now the weapons were much bigger (up to 800 times more powerful than the Hiroshima bomb), more plentiful, and more accurate. It was a straightforward task, working with physicists, epidemiologists, radiation experts, and trauma specialists, but this time we did the calculations city by city, in what we called "the bombing run." For every major city, we constructed bulls-eye grids demarcating the concentric zones of destruction resulting from a relatively modest 1-megaton airburst. And then we traveled — to New York, Baltimore, Philadelphia, Washington, Atlanta, Chicago, St. Louis, Minneapolis, Denver, San Francisco, Los Angeles, Seattle, and many cities in between — organizing public meetings and television programs, making films, debating military hawks and civil defense officials, and always showing the local bulls-eye of destruction. As PSR grew, its physician-members learned to lobby Congress in support of arms control legislation. The central message was always the same: physicians had a responsibility to use their

skills to inform the public — in a democracy, the ultimate ar-
biters of policy.

At the same time, Dr. Lown and a Soviet cardiologist
formed International Physicians for the Prevention of Nuclear
War (IPPNW), with PSR as its American affiliate. This global
federation of physicians was similarly committed to public
education about the consequences of employing these weapons of mass destruction. In 1985, IPPNW was awarded the
Nobel Prize for Peace; as national president-elect of PSR, I
attended the ceremonies in Oslo. One year later I was in Russia, leading a PSR delegation to examine the victims of the
terrifying nuclear plant explosion at Chernobyl and reporting,
first hand, on the medical and environmental consequences.

With the collapse of the Soviet Union and the end of the
cold war, PSR's work is far from done. The world is still awash
in nuclear weapons, and now we are beginning to confront
the enormous environmental contamination resulting from
their production. A PSR task force has critically examined the
Department of Energy's epidemiologic studies of its own nuclear weapons workforce — a classic case of the fox guarding
the chicken coop — and its bland assurances of safety. We are
working to end the unwarranted secrecy that had, for decades,
thrown a false blanket of "national security" over the relevant
cancer and environmental data, as if the public health were
too sensitive to be shared with the public. Now we are turning
our attention to a wide range of environmental health issues
in the United States and internationally.

In 1986, a Boston physician, Dr. Jonathan Fine, convened a group of physicians to apply their skills to another
problem: the violations of human rights and international humanitarian law that attend virtually every armed conflict,
civil war, so-called "low-intensity war," and internal struggle
against a repressive government. Torture, violations of medical neutrality (the sanctity of hospitals and health workers),
the murder of innocent noncombatants, the violation of the
rights of the sick and wounded to health care, systematic

rape, assaults on children, interference with humanitarian relief, and the use of indiscriminate weapons (nerve and mustard gases, land mines) all were common.

The group became a national organization, Physicians for Human Rights (PHR), and it established the unique usefulness of medical skills in the investigation, documentation, and prevention of human rights violations. In more than 40 missions to some 35 countries, PHR has sent teams representing every discipline — internal medicine, pediatrics, trauma medicine, surgery, forensic pathology and anthropology, epidemiology, psychiatry, environmental medicine, toxicology, and others — into the field. They have documented the use of poison gas against the Kurds of Iraq and dissidents in former Soviet Georgia; the devastating effects of land mines in Cambodia, Somalia, and El Salvador; mass executions, systematic rape, and assaults on civilians in the former Yugoslavia; violations of medical neutrality in Haiti, Thailand and the Kashmir; and torture in almost every country, including some prisons in the United States. To me, this work is an international extension of the struggle for civil rights at home and confirmation of the belief that the dignity and rights of the individual are intrinsic to medicine.

And in a larger sense, these "crusades" are simply an extension of the work of social and community medicine, a discipline that has never restricted itself to the lecture hall and campus. They express the same core values and use many of the same methodological tools as the discipline itself.

The last few years have brought other forms of return to earlier roots. In the Delta, after years of deficit, decline, and nepotism, the Department of Health and Human Services demanded the election of a new and representative Board and transferred control of the health center back to the people it served. In my former job of Executive Director is Dr. L. C. Dorsey, a remarkable civil rights worker who joined the health center staff in 1967, served as director of the farm cooperative, and subsequently earned a doctoral degree in social work. The

health center, in a new and much larger building, is flourish-
ing, and a satellite center has been opened in Greenville,
where it all began in 1964. Aware of the dozens of studies
demonstrating that health centers increase access to care, reduce hospitalizations, and are uniquely responsive to the communities they serve, the Clinton administration plans to
increase national funding and restore some of the vital services — outreach, health education, and environmental medicine — that were cut in the 1980s. John Hatch and I return
often. We have been taping interviews with the early community leaders and local staff members, many of them now quite
old, who helped launch and shape the whole enterprise. Some
day, we hope, there will be time to write the whole history.

There is yet another closing of the circle. In South Africa,
one of the important embattled organizations fighting apartheid was the National Medical and Dental Association
(NAMDA), a multiracial group of health workers who defied
the racist government's edicts, struggled to improve health
care for nonwhites, documented the health consequences of
brutal segregation and inequity in the townships and so-
called black homelands, and provided medical care and protection for protestors and prisoners. An American support
group, the Committee for Health in Southern Africa, was
formed under the leadership of Mervyn Susser, a South
African political exile and distinguished epidemiologist at
Columbia University's Faculty of Medicine. In 1989, after
years of visa denials and 32 years after my first visit as a
medical student, I returned to South Africa. My trip was part
of a mission organized by the American Association for the
Advancement of Science to document the health consequences
of apartheid.

A few years later, after the release of Nelson Mandela,
I returned again to help plan the country's first school of public health at the University of the Western Cape. On one of
those visits, I met an accomplished pediatrician, a Zulu
woman who had returned after fleeing into political exile as

an African National Congress activist. I asked where she had been born. "Polela," she said, and it turned out we had met before, when she was a young child and one of my patients at the health center. The meeting gave me a chance to ask if a story I had heard was true: that the miserably poor region served by the health center — an area of eroded land, thatched huts, hunger, and few schools — had produced an extraordinary number of professionals and political activists, even after the health center had been closed by the apartheid regime. The physician herself was clearly one of those. "Yes," she said, "but not from the whole tribal reserve. You had to live near the health center to see the programs and the role models, but you also had to live near the highway."

That seemed to make no sense. "Why the highway?" I asked. "Because," she said, "you had to *really* understand that there was a road out."

It seems to me that a central task of medicine is not merely to treat illness but to help provide a road out of the conditions — poverty, unemployment, lack of educational opportunity, dangerous physical and biological environments — that greatly increase risk. In short, medicine must bring about change in the social order. Most students come to the profession, I think, for reasons beyond their specific interests in treatment or research or the intellectual challenges or the one-on-one emotional rewards. They want to make the world a better place. In the 19th century, when medicine had much less to offer, the connection between social circumstance and the inequitable distribution of disease was much easier to see. There is so much knowledge now to master, and mastering it is so important, that larger visions can be lost. A few pages back, I called this work my salvation, in the sense that I need it for personal fulfillment, for the feeling of deep and unquestioning satisfaction that comes when work is an expression of one's central values. But I would not argue for a moment that social and community medicine is the only choice, somehow better than others, or that those who follow other paths in medicine are somehow missing out or lacking in social concern.

Every choice has its gains and losses. For me, the biggest loss was to depart from clinical medicine, which I loved — but this course was the only responsible one once the burdens of project direction, grant writing, and social campaigning made it impossible to stay current in clinical knowledge. This is a common dilemma among workers in community medicine and public health. My fondest fantasy is that on retirement I will reverse the usual sequence, find someplace that will give an old man a year or two of refresher residency, and return to practice. There were other lessons along the way: one is to value family, given a second chance. (There is a wonderful line in the 1960s musical *Hair* that runs, "Never mind the bleeding crowd; I need a friend.") Another lesson is that of distinguishing between moral outrage, the central fuel of social commitment, and an overbearing self-righteousness, the fuel of intolerant zealots.

The gains? These include lifelong friends from Mississippi, South Africa, Harlem, the West Bank and Gaza Strip, China, Russia, Boston, Yugoslavia, Israel, Tanzania, Chile, and elsewhere, all of whom had much to teach me; continuing exposure to inhumanity, personal and social brutality, and oppression — a gain because it makes indifference impossible; coming in contact with people living lives of remarkable courage and integrity; the direct, tangible sense of making a difference, building institutions, and influencing public policy by convincing the public.

The editors of this volume have asked for recommendations for involving other physicians in similar work — work that is possible, part-time and intermittently, for doctors in every field, as exemplified by the many physicians who left their practices to help out in Mississippi or go on PHR missions or work for organizations like PSR. For them, as for those who might choose such work full-time, it seems to me,

the recommendation is the same: Watch for the moment —
the opportunity — that reflects your values. Seize it.

POSTSCRIPT

Dr. H. Jack Geiger continues to teach as the Arthur C.
Logan Professor of Community Medicine at the City University of New York Medical School. He is the immediate past
president and board member of Physicians for Human Rights,
a board member of Physicians for Social Responsibility, and
president of the Committee for Health in Southern Africa.
For 1 month each year, he serves as Mary Weston Trust Visiting Professor at the University of Natal Medical School in
Durban, South Africa.

CHAPTER III

AN ADVOCATE IN ASIA

JUDITH LONGSTAFF MACKAY

In 1993, a smokers' rights group in the United States described me as "psychotic human garbage, a gibbering Satan, an insane psychotic just like Hitler, using fatuous, smarmy drivel and distortions, and diatribes full of putrid corruption, lies, conspiracy, and total censorship." They concluded by stating that I was "devoid of any sanity, any morality, or any human-being-ness of any kind," was "nothing more than an evil-possessed, power-lusting piece of meat," and they threatened to "utterly destroy" me.

My job? Working to reduce the appalling toll tobacco takes worldwide. Currently, tobacco contributes to 3 million deaths a year, a figure expected to rise to 10 million by the year 2025. Because the burden of this epidemic has shifted from rich to poor countries, most of my work is in developing countries in the Asia Pacific region.

So how does someone born and brought up in a small village on the northeast coast of England end up working as a health advocate on tobacco control in countries such as

China and Mongolia and provoking such diatribes from the international tobacco companies and their supporters?

Little predicted such a future. Until I went to medical school, I lived with my parents and grandparents, attended a local school, and rarely traveled out of England. But seeds were being sown, and I can look back on childhood influences that shaped my life. My mother most certainly transmitted a fighting spirit (which persists in her as she approaches 90 years). My mother has always said that because of the large difference in age between my older sister and me, she brought up "two only children." She remembers me as a headstrong child who was, in fact, quite difficult to bring up. Perhaps my dislike of people imposing authority over me started at a very early age.

My parents provided a stable, supportive, and caring environment. My mother was 38 and my father nearing 50 years at the time of my birth, and we lived with my grandparents in a three-generational household. Thus, I was brought up in a rather old-fashioned, Victorian way, where parents and other adults did not discuss feelings or communicate with children at a personal or intimate level. I have no recollection, for example, of anyone ever asking me about my feelings. I now think that much of my behavior in childhood resulted from the fact that I was never taught to understand myself. I realize that I was not a "bad" child, but I was rather lonely and confused as to how to deal with myself and with the world. I have often wondered if the component of my work that puts me in the public limelight is, at least in part, related to an innate need for recognition and approval.

I am very much like my mother in temperament, so we often sparked each other off. I have now learned to appreciate all that she did for me, and we communicate more openly, closely, and straightforwardly. My mother is now almost 90 years old. If the tobacco industry could see her now, and witness her spirit, they really would be worried!

I never met anyone who didn't like my father. He was one of nature's gentlemen — kind and courteous — yet he never suffered fools gladly. My father went to sea in 1912 when he was only 15 years old, and spent his whole life in the merchant navy. He was away at sea for all but a few weeks each year. In fact, because of World War II, we were apart until I was almost 2 years old. In 1941, when his ship was requisitioned and used as a troop carrier, he successfully evacuated 4000 British, Australian, and other troops from Greece under heavy bombardment despite pitch darkness and the absence of charts.

For his bravery in saving the lives of so many men, my father was awarded the Distinguished Service Cross, a decoration usually reserved for military people in the Royal Navy. He once had a ship torpedoed under him and had to take to the rafts when he was traveling to Africa to take up a new command. He and five others bobbed on the sea for more than 24 hours before being fortuitously saved by a rescue ship during their final sweep for survivors.

His was always described as a "happy ship." On the job, he was a strict but fair disciplinarian, highly regarded by all who worked with him. He had an extensive knowledge, respect, and love for the sea (which I have inherited) and an uncanny ability to "read" the sea's moods that comes from years on the bridge. As a senior captain, he passed advanced exams in navigation and radar, exams that other senior captains failed; from my father I inherited an interest in technology (including my current passion for computers). As he did, I always take my work very seriously and study with commitment.

At home he was a calm, gentle, and kind man, a good complement to my mother's more dynamic personality. In his quiet manner, he was as supportive of my career as was my mother. As the years go by, I believe I increasingly exhibit his quieter qualities.

Standing up for principles runs far back in the family. My mother came from a Victorian, Methodist background and

was one of three children, the only girl. Even at the turn of
the century, my grandfather sternly believed in equal education for girls. My mother had to translate Latin prose every
single night for my grandfather, although for some curious
reason neither of her brothers had to undergo this strict discipline. Without question, my mother was encouraged —
indeed, was expected — to go to university, and she joined
one of the first groups of women ever to do so. My grandfather's dedication to equal educational opportunities for girls,
my mother's strength of character, my father's loyal encouragement, and my own subsequent involvement with the
women's movement in the 1970s were major influences contributing to my role in tobacco control.

At university my mother developed an inherited form of
deafness, otosclerosis, and, embarrassed by the enormous bat-
tery pack for her hearing aid, she did not take up a professional
career. My mother's sole occupation as a homemaker, however,
did not prevent her from encouraging me without question to
undertake the lengthy medical course at the University of Edinburgh in Scotland. Edinburgh was renowned for training
more women than most universities, but even so fewer than
one-quarter of the medical students were women. After graduation in 1966, at 22 years of age, I stayed in Edinburgh and
worked with Sir John Crofton, one of the earliest pioneers exploring the link between tobacco and ill health. He planted the
seeds of awareness about tobacco's destructive effects in me
and became my life-long mentor, supporter, and friend.

It was while working with Sir John in the City Hospital
in Edinburgh that I met my future husband, a Scottish doctor
on study leave from Hong Kong. Married in Edinburgh, I became a "camp follower," moving immediately after my intern
year and registration to Hong Kong, which has been my home
for more than half my life. Camp follower I did not remain
for long.

I arrived in Hong Kong at an interesting time (and shall
probably leave at an interesting time, as sovereignty passes

back from Britain to China in 1997). Hong Kong is located on China's southern coast, and almost 99% of the population is Chinese. Although its administration will remain colonial until 1997, an increasing number of civil servants are Chinese, many of whom hold senior positions.

Back in 1967, China's Cultural Revolution had spilled over into Hong Kong, with Red Guards brandishing Mao's "little red book" and shouting anti-British slogans on the streets. Bomb scares occurred daily, and the Communist banks and schools were barricaded with barbed wire. We learned to avoid abandoned packages in the streets and to endure the constant wails of police sirens. But, resilient as ever, Hong Kong emerged to establish itself as an international financial and business center, a far cry from my first memories of a rather sleepy town disrupted by bombs.

Incredibly, in spite of my family background, I bought into a nonfeminist philosophy that I would never "work" again. With a doctor–husband, what was the need? It was Hong Kong's beaches for me. This may have been partly a reaction to my strenuous intern year, and it only lasted a few weeks. Medical jobs were almost impossible to obtain for non-Cantonese speakers, so I enrolled in a language school and mastered colloquial and medical Cantonese. Never one with an ear for languages, I found this very difficult, but it was essential in enabling me to continue professional work in "Western medicine" (as opposed to the traditional Chinese medicine, acupuncture, and herbalism still very popular in Hong Kong).

My first paid job in Hong Kong politicized and radicalized me in a totally unexpected way. I answered a job advertisement to discover, at the interview, that the advertised salary was for a male doctor. In conformity with Hong Kong government practice, the salary for a female doctor would be 75% of the advertised "male" salary. I then realized why black boxes appeared around two job advertisements in the *British Medical Journal* — those in South Africa because of racial discrimination and those in Hong Kong because of sexual discrimination in pay. This was my first recognition of sexual discrimination, and I was outraged, truly outraged. Gritting my teeth, I took the job, but I failed to earn equal pay for another few years.

In 1969 and 1970 I gave birth to our two sons. The next few years were spent doing part-time research with the Paediatric Department of Hong Kong University. Here, I immersed myself in children's growth and development, contributing to a study unique at that time.

Many aspects of the family-versus-career dilemma were not a dilemma for me. I realized in early adulthood that I would never be content living my life through another person — being somebody's wife or somebody's mother. I have always had a strong need for independence, a need to be myself and to be judged for myself. I probably would have resented any person to whom, by imposition of will or circumstance, I had abrogated my self.

I have also been fortunate in having paid domestic help. I now have a very straightforward attitude toward employing a person to do this job for me — I employ domestic help in the matter-of-fact way that I would employ a secretary or a nurse. Having all the cooking, cleaning, and washing done has given me time that I (and my husband) would otherwise not have had. Domestic help has certainly been an enabling factor in my life.

Yet my main difficulty still was lack of time — I was always juggling so many roles. When the children were young, in particular, I felt terribly stretched; sometimes I felt I would crack if I had to meet just one more demand. I felt that I was juggling several different jobs and coping with myriad responsibilities. I tried to become superefficient and set myself standards that were hard to live up to, but I am certain that I was a better mother for having an interesting job and a sense of self. Our sons, now adults, escape guilt trips. They know that I am busy, happy, fulfilled, and glad to see them when we can — it is a very straight-forward relationship.

I have been married since 1967. My husband weathered, with equanimity, my considerable transformation from the Yorkshire girl he married to a committed feminist and out-spoken health advocate. He is a quiet and gentle man with a tremendous sense of humor that has grown over the years. He is not at all fazed by the fact that I am very much in the public eye and that many people ask him "Are you Judith Mackay's husband?" He has given me nothing but total and loyal support and is like a safe harbor for me when I return home weary from battles with the tobacco companies and nonstop traveling. My husband remains my best friend, my support, my oasis.

My husband is like my father — everyone likes him. He was always courteous and considerate with his patients. At a recent dinner given by his medical colleagues, one of the other doctors said that John was unique in the practice: in 30 years, there had not been one single complaint about him from fellow doctors, patients, nurses, or anyone else.

His colleague amused everyone by reading a 1963 letter of recommendation for the post in Hong Kong from a Con-sultant Neurosurgeon in Edinburgh:

> I have nothing but praise for Dr. Mackay, as he was most assiduous in carrying out all his duties in the Depart-ment. His clinical abilities in examination and writing case notes are high, and he has a pleasant personality and was extremely popular with his patients and the nursing, medical and rehabilitation staffs. He is intelli-gent and very interested in clinical medicine with a par-ticular bent towards neurology and psychiatry.

My husband was always helpful with the children when they were young, but, in spite of the relative equality of our marriage, I still somehow had prime responsibility for the children, the house and our social program.

Both of our sons were born and grew up in Hong Kong. They returned to Scotland for their final years of schooling, then went to Cambridge University in England. After 3 years of premed at Cambridge, our elder son Andrew (born 1969) went to Glasgow University in Scotland for his clinical courses and graduated in 1993. I see much of my own temperament reflected in him as he grows up.

Our younger son Richard (born 1970) graduated with a degree in Environmental Sciences, which he is augmenting with studies in Environmental Law and Management. He is much more like his father, inheriting both his sense of humor and his quiet sense of self. Both of our sons are nonsmokers!

My early brush with pay discrimination led to my involvement in the early 1970s with the women's movement, which in several ways moved me closer to my present career. My commitment to my career solidified, influenced by a chance remark by an older American woman at one of the feminist meetings. She said that as I had two children and could expect to live until the age of 80 years or more, the major part of my life — even if I spent 15 years away from my profession for child rearing — would not be spent in child rearing. For the first time in my life, I seriously addressed long-term career options. After 6 years away from hospital medicine, I dedicated the next 3 years to a training program in internal medicine in the Medical Faculty at the University of Hong Kong. These years culminated in multiple examinations to obtain Membership (then subsequently Fellowship) in the Royal College of Physicians of the United Kingdom. I then worked as a specialist in internal medicine in a government-supported university hospital for the next decade, teaching medical students and establishing training programs for postgraduate doctors and other medical staff. Without exception, all our junior doctors passed their British postgraduate specialty exams.

After feminism, hospital work became the second major route to my becoming a tobacco control advocate. The Hong

Kong government estimated that over 3000 deaths were caused annually from tobacco smoking (out of a population of 6 million), making it the largest preventable cause of death. On a more personal level, my work on the medical wards was almost completely related to the end results of smoking. Although occasionally a nonsmoking youth with typhoid or tuberculosis would come in, there was a general maxim on the male medical ward that we "never admitted a nonsmoker." Cancer, heart disease, stroke, and chronic bronchitis — all tobacco related — were our most common admissions. Dealing daily with incurable lung, heart, and other smoking-related diseases, I came to feel my work was a patch-and-repair job. So many of these diseases were irreversible, even with expensive technology, that I realized that the overall health of Hong Kong's population would never improve unless there was an appropriate emphasis on prevention. Increasingly, I felt the urge to move into this field.

Concurrently, my involvement with feminist issues led me to an interest in womens' health, with its emphasis on educating women about their bodies and how they work and promoting self-help and participation in health care decisions. In 1972, I helped found the International Feminist League, an organization comprised largely of expatriate women and principally devoted to personal growth. Through consciousness-raising groups we explored relationships, family, our bodies, work, media representation of women, health, and health care.

My focus on women's issues transformed my thoughts and actions, which did not lie easily with many of my friends, male and female alike. On the one hand, I felt the excitement of immense personal growth, but on the other, I felt a sense of loss as friends found my growth and the independence it brought too threatening for comfort.

Surprisingly, there were very few female role models or mentors in my professional life. Virtually all the decisionmakers working in hospital medicine in Hong Kong were men;

in hospital medicine I was the only woman and the only foreigner in a department of 25 doctors. The same ratios applied globally in tobacco control, with rare exceptions such as Dr. Eileen Crofton in Scotland, Professor Ruth Roemer in Los Angeles, and Professor Li Wan Xian in Shanghai. Thus, I identified with women but worked with men. Even today, there are only a handful of women in Asia who are active at the national level in tobacco control policy, and in the mid-1990s, I still usually find myself the only woman on senior committees, plenary sessions at conferences and government advisory bodies. In light of this situation, I spend a lot of time proposing women's names for appropriate committees and conferences, and trying to bring the issue of smoking by women to its rightful place of importance. So although I myself have never had the benefit of a role model, I hope that I provide such a model for others, and that the path is less lonely for women who follow.

It was from the women's movement that I learned political and media lobbying, which served me well when I took on the powerful tobacco barons. Joining older, well-educated Chinese women, my first campaign was to abolish the concubine law, which stated that a man could legally have many wives but that a woman could have only one husband. This law had been abolished 20 years earlier in China as one of the first acts of Mao Zedong's new regime. In Hong Kong, however, it was still in place, principally because many of our legislators had concubines and thus had a clear disinterest in changing the status quo! The new law was made nonretrospective so that older women officially recognized as legal concubines, whose children were legitimate, and who had legal rights to the husband's estate, would suffer no reverse.

I then became involved in successful campaigns for separate taxation for married women, equal pay and terms of service for married women in the civil service, and maternity leave. We also worked on behalf of victims of child abuse and rape and established a refuge for battered women. All these

issues were extremely controversial at the time, as it was commonly (and erroneously) believed that physical abuse did not
occur in Chinese families. Learning when to confront, when
to cooperate, when to deal with issues quietly, and when to
go public — all these skills were invaluable assets when I became a health advocate. Although it took time, I also learned
not to allow strident and personal criticism to affect me when
I was campaigning for something I believed in.

Although I lobbied for a wide range of legislation, I became most involved with women's health issues, including re-
productive health, health at work, mental health, cancer,
nutrition, exercise, and smoking. My association with these
issues led to an invitation to do a regular 2-hour weekly live
program on women's health on the government radio channel.
The programs quickly became renowned in Hong Kong for
dealing with personal health problems in an extremely frank
and straightforward manner. The Director of Broadcasting
feared losing his job when he heard the show hostess and
me discussing sexuality on air, a taboo subject in Hong Kong
in the 1970s. I had said that, unlike men's familiarity with
their genitalia, and in contrast to women's frequent examination of their faces, some women had never seen their own
clitoris and vulva. I suggested that women use a small mirror
and gave hints on how they might recognize physical land-
marks. During the next few days, there was a run on hand
mirrors in the colony, which were by then all sold out! The
Director of Broadcasting need not have worried; the show became extremely popular, and we were inundated with calls
each week.

But my life's voyage ran into rapids more turbulent than
my wildest dreams. My difficulties began when I started writing a 2-year series on women's health for Hong Kong's leading
English-language newspaper. I wrote not only as a health professional but also, having experienced childbirth and used con-
traception, as a female consumer. Thus, I did not write "when
your doctor tells you to have a hysterectomy" but "when you

and your doctor decide a hysterectomy is necessary." This promotion of the shifting of power in the doctor–patient relationship did not please some of my medical colleagues, especially those used to patient acquiescence. One day a prominent gynecologist (who was large in size) came to the hospital, backed me up against a wall in a most intimidating manner, and told me that my newspaper series "had to stop." He said that doctors did not like it and that I should know that I had some "enemies in very high places." The trigger for this incident had occurred earlier that day, when a patient questioned the doctor after she was fitted with an intrauterine contraceptive device (the patient had asked if the device was copper). He then asked if she had been reading Judith Mackay's column, and when she said "yes," he hit the roof, telling her that whether it was copper or not was "none of her business." Such was the attitude of some members of Hong Kong's medical establishment in the 1970s.

Although I was shaken by this incident, worse was still to come. Hoping to prevent any ethical problems, I had written to the Medical Council (the government-appointed regulatory and disciplinary body for doctors) only to be told they would not give advice. Shortly afterwards, I was informed that a doctor had complained to the Medical Council, charging that my newspaper series constituted advertising. This was a truly bizarre accusation, as the newspaper and I had agreed on basic ethics: that the paper would use my married name of Mackay rather than my professional name, would not state where I worked, my position, or the type of job I did, and would publish a regular rejoinder that I could not see or correspond with any readers in a professional capacity. Indeed, overwhelmed by patients in a public hospital, the last thing I or the hospital wanted was more patients. The 600-bed hospital served a poor district of 750,000 people, so our acute wards and intensive care unit were incredibly busy. My patients neither spoke English nor knew me by my English name of Longstaff; they all called me by my Chinese name of Dr. Lung (Dr. Dragon!). Many were illiterate; certainly none were readers of the English-language *South China Morning Post*.

Found guilty of professional misconduct on the charge of advertising by an all-male board of Medical Council doctors, I took the case to the Appeals Court, which gave a landmark ruling in my favor. All charges were dismissed, and I was awarded costs (the opposition had to pay all my legal fees), a sure indication of my innocence. When it became public knowledge that I had endured a year of hearings, it caused a public uproar. The editor of the *South China Morning Post* said that during his 26 years as editor, his paper had never received more letters on any topic.

The case was the first successful appeal against the Medical Council in Hong Kong's history and was written up in law journals in Hong Kong and elsewhere. The editorial in the *Hong Kong Law Journal* noted with surprise that the Council had refused to give advice when I had asked, ending with the diplomatic but penetrating comment that reduction of the secrecy surrounding cases like mine (such as the Medical Council's refusal — even to this day — to identify the complainant and its refusal to publish its reasons for its decision) would "minimize the widespread suspicions that it occasionally disciplines practitioners to discourage the expression of views displeasing to the medical establishment."

I appealed the case for very practical reasons. I was determined to continue in health education but faced the prospect of being struck off the Medical Register. The legal ruling became an important precedent for doctors who wished to appear in public, in relation to either health issues or political and social activities. I knew that the Medical Council verdict was manifestly wrong, and this episode, although painful to this day, taught me to stand up for principles and not to be cowed or silenced by powerful organizations.

By coincidence, the very day the Appeals Court ruled in my favor, Ivan Illich, the author of *Medical Nemesis* and *The*

Limits of Medicine, happened to be in Hong Kong. Using
Dr. Illich's analytical framework, an academic from the University of Hong Kong wrote that "Judith Mackay is seen [by
the medical profession] to be guilty of . . . 'demythologizing'
medicine." Demands for explanation by patients, they wrote,
threaten doctors' power, prestige, and income. By supplying
health information, they continued, I was placing health care
back into the hands of the sufferer, undermining the medical
profession's control of all events related to illness and health.

In an ironic postscript, a few years later I received an
honor from the British Queen, becoming a Member of the
Order of the British Empire (MBE). For me, this award "for
services to health education in Hong Kong since 1967" finally
vindicated my fervent (and truly innocent) commitment to
health education.

Through writing the series on women's health, I came to
some new realizations. Most striking was that although
women's health programs traditionally address gynecological
issues, more women die from smoking than from all methods
of birth control combined. In addition, girls and women are
both exploited and aggressively recruited by tobacco companies, whose advertisements feature attractive, slim, successful women. Cigarette ads promise emancipation, whereas in
reality smoking is yet another form of bondage for women.
My reaction to these tactics formed the basis for a series of
articles on women and tobacco. The violent response to these
articles marked a personal turning point, one of those single
events that change one's life.

One of the transnational cigarette companies published
a booklet claiming that the "anti-smoking lobby in Hong Kong
is largely anonymous, unidentifiable, entirely unrepresentative and unaccountable." In contrast, the self-promotional
booklet claimed "the tobacco industry comprises identifiable,
legal, accountable, commercial organizations." This booklet,
denying the health evidence ("it has not been proven that
these illnesses are actually caused by smoking") and claiming

to be an "important source of reliable information," so enraged me that from that moment on, I worked on tobacco control, abandoning curative hospital medicine in 1984.

At first it was a lonely existence. Then support came from one cancer doctor in Hong Kong, followed by governmental support from one of the finest senior civil servants it has been my pleasure to know. Tobacco control advocates from around the world gradually made contact, and I, in turn, have managed to establish networks throughout Asia.

Even in the early days, the battles with the tobacco industry were tough, and every step of legislation fiercely challenged. Hong Kong assumed an importance far beyond its population of only 6 million; all the tobacco companies base their regional offices in Hong Kong, which straddles the crossroads of Asia and serves as the gateway to China. I provoked further resentment by widely disseminating information on Hong Kong's successful tobacco control measures, giving rise to a domino effect of similar legislation in the region.

The tobacco industry attacked journalists who wrote articles on smoking, claiming to their editors that "the use of pictures of cancerous lungs clearly attempts to suggest, without any foundation, that the disease was caused by smoking, and is highly irresponsible in its appeal to emotional and sensational instincts." Public relations firms that helped with events such as the annual Smoke-Out Day claimed they were unable to help us any more.

My indignation about foreign cigarette companies' treatment of Asia gained momentum in 1986, when I attended a major tobacco industry exhibition in Hong Kong. Identifying myself as a medical doctor, I asked one of the representatives manning a U.S. tobacco export booth if smoking's harmfulness troubled her. Her male colleague overheard the question and sidled up to answer: "It's OK, although we grow all our tobacco in the U.S.A., we don't sell any there; we export it all. Only Asians smoke it." I was flabbergasted at this callous, racist remark. The representatives were more than a little taken aback by my sweetly delivered reply: "Many of us in Asia would find those remarks extremely offensive."

There were, however, many amusing incidents. The Broadcasting Review Board held public hearings in 1985 to discuss, *inter alia,* whether or not to ban tobacco advertising on television in Hong Kong. During these proceedings, a Tobacco Institute press release quoted me as saying, in relation to tobacco advertising, that "nobody is saying that a ban would have any effect." Incensed, I realized that the industry had lifted a few words from a longer sentence: "Nobody is saying that a ban, completely unsupported by any other measures, will *alone* have a dramatic effect upon smoking rates."

That day, I encouraged our two sons to attend the hearings to hear tobacco executives first hand. Although they had often heard me speak about smoking, the testimony of the cigarette company executives filled them with such indignation that I believe they became confirmed nonsmokers from that moment on. I was seated in the official area, and clearly the tobacco executives did not realize that these two teenagers in the public gallery were in any way connected with me. The boys overheard the Philip Morris team discussing me personally and professionally in words such as the boys had never heard before (and which are quite unrepeatable here!).

Other fun episodes came when the General Manager of British American Tobacco, who had lobbied intensely at the hearings, was transferred in 1986 from Hong Kong to Malaysia. A newspaper report announced his departure with the heading "Tobacco man goes out blazing." It described his farewell skit, a message for the Chairman of the Broadcasting Review Board: "Could the advertising power of this man make you eat kangaroo stew?" a play on the Chairman's name (Power), his nationality (Australian), and the idea that advertising would never induce anyone to take up a new habit. I responded in verse (as I was to do many times from then on):

Ad with a power of persuasion

"Tobacco man goes out (a)blazing"
Leaves a question for all to pursue:
"Could the advertising power of this man
Make you eat kangaroo stew?"

Now kangaroo stew I've not heard of
To a Brit it is something quite new
But the power of the ad is upon me
I want to try kangaroo stew

It's not that I'm changing the roo brand
Or switching from dingo fondue
A thought in my mind has been planted
To sample this kangaroo stew

Ads say the sophisticates like it
The rich and the powerful too
What attraction this product does offer
This wonderful kangaroo stew

I could tame a wild horse if I ate it
Brave rapids in just a canoe
Land the man of my dreams with no effort
All is promised by kangaroo stew

Alas Gordon Watson has left us
Disappeared in a puff of smoke blue
Perhaps to persuade the Malaysians
To take up this kangaroo stew

Those familiar with tobacco advertisements immediately recognized the popular advertising images, but people who had not seen the earlier article about the tobacco man's departure were most puzzled as to why I had penned a verse about kangaroo stew!

Some of the battles had clandestine aspects. In 1986, a go-between phoned to tell me that a "Deep Throat" associated with U.S. Tobacco had informed him of a plan to imminently launch smokeless tobacco (sucking, chewing tobacco, and snuff) in Hong Kong. To this day I do not know the identification of "Deep Throat," not even whether it is a she or a he. Immediately, I contacted the Hong Kong government and helped plan a "preemptive strike," a ban on import, manufacture, and sale of smokeless tobacco products before they became established on the market.

As soon as the government announced the proposed ban, "enquiries" were received by individual United States Senators, the Commercial Officer of the U.S. Consulate, U.S. Tobacco, and a leading law firm in Hong Kong. These inquiries were hardly neutral. Questions asked by the U.S. Consulate included: On what basis had Hong Kong decided on the ban? Had there been any documents from the U.S. Surgeon General? Could he see copies of World Health Organization and Department of Health and Human Services correspondence? (The answer was no, these were confidential.) Inquiries notwithstanding, the government introduced legislation to implement the ban in early 1987.

Although U.S. Tobacco claimed that it did not sell to children under 18 years of age, we recruited three 13- and 14-year-old school children, equipped them with hidden microphones, and sent them to outlets carrying smokeless tobacco products. All three bought the product unhindered, and none were asked their ages or issued warnings. Although the children initially were nervous, they felt angry about how easily they had purchased smokeless tobacco and felt a sense of importance when their report was submitted to government.

But there were more political pressures to come, in the shape of a letter from U.S. Senators Robert Dole, Christopher Dodd, Bob Kasten, and Lowell P. Weicker, Jr., to the Hong Kong government: "We believe (a ban) would (be viewed in the United States as) an unfair and discriminatory restriction on foreign trade . . ." They continued that the ban could cause "a potential barrier to our people's historic trade relationship" — words to make any trading partner tremble. Not all U.S.

government officials behaved this way. Henry Waxman, the Chairman of Senate Health Subcommittee, and the U.S. Surgeon General, Dr. C. Everett Koop, as well as many other health professionals gave firm support to Hong Kong.

The ban went through, and Hong Kong became the second place in the world and the first in Asia to ban smokeless tobacco. Despite their knowledge of tobacco industry tactics, government officials reported feeling stunned by the fierce political pressures they had had to withstand.

Hong Kong's government also became the first in Asia to establish and fund a tobacco control agency. In 1987, I was appointed the founding Executive Director of the Hong Kong Council on Smoking and Health, popularly known as COSH. Over the next 2 years, battles grew even more heated as new regulatory legislation was introduced and implemented. Today, Hong Kong vies with Singapore for having the lowest prevalence of smoking in the world; it is no coincidence that these two governments have firmly grasped the political nettle of tobacco control. For me, working within Hong Kong's political system was useful for subsequent work with other governments in Asia, where the "top-down" approach is the principal route.

Increasingly, I was overwhelmed by requests for assistance from neighboring Asian countries. In 1989, I resigned from COSH to establish the Asian Consultancy on Tobacco Control, a coordinating organization that facilitates the sharing of information, experience, and expertise on tobacco control among countries in the Asia–Pacific region.

Overall, 60–70% of men and 2–10% of women in Asia are daily smokers. The number of smokers is rising as a result of population expansion, greater independence and affluence among youth, increased smoking among girls, and lack of funds for tobacco control. The tobacco industry itself has predicted a 33% increase in sales between 1991 and 2000. In fact, the Western Pacific Region is the *only* World Health Organization (WHO) region where per-capita tobacco consumption is rising. There are no data on how much the tobacco industry spends on advertising and promotion in Asia — this information seems to be a closely guarded secret.

Many people in the United States think that the tobacco epidemic is being conquered, but nothing could be further from the truth. The world's tobacco problem is not being solved; it is expanding in economically poor countries. Although indigenous tobacco production and consumption remain a major problem in most Asian countries, the powerful international tobacco cartel poses a particularly ominous threat. With markets slowly decreasing in the West, companies are moving in on developing countries, where huge numbers of potential smokers reside. For example, there are already 300 million smokers in China alone, more than the entire population of the United States.

With only 4% of the world's population it would hardly matter if every smoker in the United States quit, provided that the 60% of Asian men who already smoke local tobacco could be persuaded to switch to foreign cigarettes, and if significant numbers of women could be persuaded to take up the habit. "What do we want?" asked a tobacco executive recently. "We want Asia." This was spelled out explicitly in an article entitled "Bright Future Predicted for Asia Pacific" using subheadings such as "Growth Potential" and "More Smokers" in the industry journal *World Tobacco.*

Not everyone views these predictions with such enthusiasm. Oxford epidemiologist Richard Peto predicts that in China alone, 50 million of all the children alive today will eventually die prematurely by smoking. The current 3 million annual deaths worldwide from tobacco use will rise to 10 million by the year 2025, with 7 million of these deaths in developing countries and most of them in Asia (2 million in China alone). Probably the most important contribution to preventing noncommunicable diseases worldwide would be to prevent smoking among Asian women, of whom only 5% currently smoke. The battle lines are drawn.

In addition to denying incontrovertible health evidence, challenging responsible government action on tobacco, and draining their profits back to shareholders in the West, U.S. and British cigarette companies have adopted double standards in developing countries. They advertise in ways long banned on home turf, selling cigarettes with higher tar and no health warnings. The trade arm of the U.S. government, influenced by the powerful U.S. tobacco industry, threatens unilateral trade sanctions against countries that refuse to open their markets to foreign cigarettes or curtail their marketing.

Governments in developing countries are often preoccupied with other health problems, such as high infant mortality or infectious disease, and thus may neglect to create policy, laws, or health education programs on tobacco. In addition, these countries' lack of experience dealing with the transnational tobacco cartel renders them vulnerable to penetration and exploitation by foreign industry.

My job is therefore two-sided. On the one hand, I have published innumerable papers and have spoken at about 200 international conferences about the evolving nature of the tobacco control problem. I have also testified before government committees in exporting countries, with two simple requests: that their tobacco companies adhere, at minimum, to the same standards in developing countries as in their country of origin, and that a product as uniquely harmful as tobacco not be used as trade leverage.

But tobacco export trade to Asia is big business, and big business is very powerful. In 1988, the then U.S. Surgeon General, Dr. C. Everett Koop, invited me to speak at an Interagency Committee Meeting on "U.S. Trade Policies on Tobacco." When White House officials learned of this meeting, they forced a last-minute change of topic, told Dr. Koop not to meddle in international health, and demanded cancelation of my appearance. Too late — I was already airborne from Hong Kong. Along with others such as Mike Pertschuk of the

Advocacy Institute and Greg Connolly from Boston, I said that "regrettably" the express letter had not reached me in time to amend my talk in any way. It was a lively meeting, with Dr. Koop totally unrepentant about his responsibility to health on a global scale.

Congressional subcommittee hearings on the same issue were equally tense, with tobacco industry-funded congressmen directing extreme aggression toward me. I also worked with the British government, which in 1991 announced a moratorium on aid to British tobacco companies' activities in developing countries and pledged help to tobacco growers diversifying into other crops.

The other side of my job, mainly through the World Health Organization and the International Union Against Cancer, has been to work with governments and health organizations in Asia. Over the last few years, I have worked in China, Hong Kong, Indonesia, Japan, Laos, Malaysia, Mongolia, the Philippines, the Republic of Korea, Singapore, Taiwan, Thailand, and Vietnam. My work includes assisting countries in recognizing the scope of their tobacco problem, establishing a national tobacco control policy, and countering the tactics of the transnational tobacco companies.

My main jobs in these countries include:

- Acting as governmment advisor, principally to the Ministry of Health. In particular, I help them draft comprehensive tobacco control legislation. (I often think I am a closet law drafter!).
- Working with NGOs (nongovernmental organizations).
- Organizing and speaking at conferences and workshops.
- Participating in government hearings on tobacco issues.
- Providing the country with plentiful documentation.
- Running "How to" workshops: "How to do a prevalence survey," "How to work with the media," "How to draft

a model law," "How to give a paper," "How to chair a meeting," and so on. These courses have become immensely popular.

In summary, my job is to help developing countries get started on tobacco control. My work takes me to areas off the beaten track, such as China'a remote provinces — where I oversaw the quitting project for rural, illiterate, Chinese farmers — or the western part of Mongolia. In my experience, after 3 to 4 years of support, Asian countries competently run their own tobacco control programs, and national campaigns take on their own momentum. Thus, I liken my job to a catalyst: I inform and empower countries to get their national tobacco control efforts up and running.

The speed of action and long-term planning in some Asian countries is impressive. It took only 2 years for the Chinese government to draft, pass, and implement their first and far-reaching tobacco law in January 1992. When I asked Vietnam's Minister of Health a few years ago why his Ministry was taking so many steps in tobacco control, he replied, "Of course, we are just thinking 30 years into the future."

I write in medical journals and lecture in many other countries, such as Argentina, Australia, Canada, France, Germany, U.K., and the United States. I work closely with the World Health Organization and the International Union Against Cancer. One recent job, to give a practical example, has been to draft a 1995–1999 Action Plan on Tobacco or Health for the Western Pacific Regional Office of World Health Organization. Our Action Plan gave all countries in this region a series of yearly targets and goals, which included a "tobacco-advertising-free region by the year 2000."

Many people ask if I become daunted by the enormity of the problem of smoking in Asia. Certainly, tobacco consumption and related deaths will increase considerably in the next few decades. But you cannot allow the enormity of a problem to paralyze you, or you get absolutely nowhere.

The Chinese have an ancient saying: "It is better to light a candle than to curse the darkness." For me, the candle represents the systems that are being put into place by national governments to address the tobacco epidemic, and I believe these candles will ultimately burn out the epidemic. Another Chinese saying — "A journey of 10,000 miles begins with a single step" — illustrates a sobering reality: although the first steps in reducing the tobacco epidemic have been taken in some developing countries, there are still many miles ahead.

After years of working in tobacco control, a completely new opportunity arose in 1992. The editor of a series of Atlas books — on women, war and peace, the environment, the world — realized that no atlas on health existed. She asked me to be the author of *The State of Health Atlas,* hinging her decision on a statement I made about low-tar cigarettes. (The difference between high- and low-tar cigarettes is the difference between jumping out of a third-story window and a second-story window.) She wanted someone who could translate health statistics into imaginative images. Writing a book on health turned out to be a remarkably unhealthy activity. I spent hours past midnight hunched in front of a computer, poring over statistical documents, and I got insufficient exercise. The whole experience almost merited a warning: "Warning: Writing health books is hazardous to your health." My first obstacle was finding the data. The next creative challenge was converting 20,000 health statistics into maps and colorful pictures.

The Atlas won the 1994 BUPA "Highly Commended Prize" awarded by the British Society of Authors for books published in the U.K. in the medical atlas section. I am currently writing another atlas, *The State of Sex Atlas*.

I am always being challenged by the tobacco companies. Television and radio interviews and press articles were (and probably still are) monitored. At international conferences, even in the United States, I am filmed and recorded by people working for the tobacco industry (as are other key tobacco control activists). I know that the tobacco industry keeps files on me in countries throughout Asia. The industry frequently challenges the accuracy of my statistics, sometimes by "enquiries" to government departments. On one occasion, the government spokesperson commented to the inquirer that I was always "scrupulous with statistics" and that these exercises were a complete waste of everyone's time.

On radio and television I have found myself repudiated, interrupted, and threatened with legal action. On one radio program a tobacco industry man was so acrimonious that another industry executive apologized to me about her colleague's behavior! As mentioned earlier, the tobacco industry and its supporters have described me over the years as "sanctimonious," "dogmatic," "pontificating," "meddlesome," "heretic," "puritanical," "hysterical," "prejudiced," and a "Nanny." They have also stated publicly that "her views are a tedious rehash of dogmatic prejudice, [and] her appointment is akin to putting a pork butcher in charge of a Jewish kitchen . . ." (I am still trying to work out what this means!). I have even been accused of having "subliminal, repressed, sexual frustration" because I cannot bear to see the "position of a cigarette in relation to the male mouth!"

Such offensive words, and the death threat mentioned previously, completely fail to either affect or divert me. I am never quite certain whether this is their standard behavior (go for the messenger when your message doesn't stand up) or an attempt to intimidate me or a ploy to cast doubt on my credibility in the minds of the listening public.

A few years ago I came to realize that tobacco was only a vehicle, albeit a very legitimate vehicle, for me to empower individuals, organizations, and governments. Through my work I would help people recognize their ability to make decisions in the interest of their own or their country's health and to realize that they can stand up to vested commercial interests. From that moment onward, the tobacco companies became, at one level, unimportant to me. Although I had never discussed my shift of thinking with anyone, within a week my new attitude prompted the tobacco companies to ask a senior government official what had happened to me, as they "could no longer get a handle" on me.

I have often been asked, both in Hong Kong and internationally, if I fear for my safety. In 1990 I learned from a leaked, confidential document published in London that the transnational tobacco industry considered me one of the three most dangerous people in the world. This was one of the best compliments I have ever received. When the BBC asked me if I were fearful about being on the tobacco companies" "Top Three Hit List," I replied that my future safety had never been more assured. If anyone found me at the bottom of Hong Kong harbor with concrete around my feet, they would now assume it was the tobacco industry until proved otherwise. In fact, I joked, the tobacco companies would probably provide me with a bodyguard just to make sure I did not step in front of a bus by mistake!

The tobacco industry has darkly warned that I have "turned a crusade into a career." Although true, the comment carries undue negative connotations. No one says accusingly that endocrinologists have "made a career out of diabetes" or that accident and emergency doctors have "made a career out of car crashes." My career moves have certainly not been motivated by financial gain. Even in the early days, I could have earned many times more by working in private practice rather than in university and government hospitals. Nowadays, although I receive expenses when I visit different countries, since 1989 I have received no salary, and I have no organizational funding.

My professional rewards come from the extremely interesting nature of my job and my gratitude that so many countries in Asia have taken steps in tobacco control. Because I am based in an area inexperienced in tobacco control, I am privileged in helping countries make quantum leaps forward, often from scratch. Until a few years ago, Singapore and Hong Kong were the only countries in Asia to have implemented significant tobacco control measures; now virtually every country in the region has some tobacco control legislation. In addition, I visit areas where few foreigners have trod and benefit from seeing countries from the inside rather than as a tourist. I have received national awards from the British, Chinese, U.S., and Thai governments for my work. The Minister of Health in China presented me with a "National Honor Award" in the Great Hall of the People in Beijing. Shortly afterwards, I received the U.S. Surgeon General's Medallion from Dr. Koop. It is unusual for nonnationals to receive either of these awards, and to receive them from both countries is truly unique.

I have been involved with other issues as diverse as corruption prevention, holistic health centers, marriage guidance, and the Hospital Authority, and I am a Justice of the Peace, visiting prisons and Vietnamese refugee camps. The seriousness of these topics has been balanced over the years by my collection of hundreds of jokes, which I am constantly being urged to publish.

I was born a life-long campaigner. My current campaign on tobacco will certainly continue, and others may well emerge. Has it been worth it? Yes. A successful campaign in preventive health can save more lives than a lifetime of hospital practice.

POSTSCRIPT

Dr. Judith Longstaff Mackay continues her work in tobacco control, offering workshops for colleagues in areas such as organizing conferences, writing press releases, and countering tobacco industry arguments. She recently finished entering her sizable library (legislation, health education programs, newspaper articles, and abtracts for 50 countries in the Asia Pacific region) onto the computer. Current activities include authoring *The State of Sex Atlas* and preliminary research on *The State of Age Atlas*. She has also just been named a Visiting Professor at the Chinese Academy of Preventive Medicine.

CHAPTER IV

CROSSROADS

LOUIS FAZEN, M.D.

I feel ashamed to pounce upon the page with a narrative that is so open, explicit, so personal. In one sense it is a vivisection, the cutting up of a living creature to see how it works, rummaging among the still-quivering flesh for its soul.

—Richard Selzer, *Raising the Dead,* 1993

"What are you doing here?" a concerned co-worker wonders out loud. I begin searching for the answer, the summary statement. I consider my upbringing, my years of high-priced education and medical training, and my comfortable life-style. Yes, I am privileged. And yes, I am privileged to work with people living in poverty. Fortunately, Sadie answers for me. "We need him here. Don't you see all those patients at the window!"

At the most basic level, I practice pediatrics in an American ghetto. Encircled by red brick high-risers in various stages of reconditioning, I watch my step crossing through the projects. The voices and beats of African-American and

Latin-American pop culture reverberate off the buildings. The tenements are full, but bare parking lots demonstrate the outer edge of economic prosperity. Occasionally a child with a knapsack of books recognizes me from the clinic. "Hey, I know you. I seen you on TV. You're Mr. Rogers!"

In our society we become defined by our labors — I work with families who live with meager financial resources. Most are either recently coming into poverty or trying to get out of it. Some have made a life of welfare dependency. They experience the same problems affecting everyone, but the condition of poverty makes resolving these problems much more difficult. In this line of work, a doctor's black bag has to include skills in acute care, public health, and preventive medicine as well as the ability to listen to personal narratives and hear cultural refrains.

My slant on life is related to issues of scarce resources, but it wasn't always that way. I grew up in one of those *Leave It to Beaver* families of the 1950s. At a time when just owning a car was the dividing line, I remember having a convertible. Our home life supported the sense of unlimited possibilities, given hard work and the requisite resources. My father and his father before him modeled the role of the master craftsmen, practicing general surgery in southeastern Wisconsin for nearly eight decades. Hard-working father and nurturing mother at home feeding seven at the dinner table: it was the best of Midwestern America. I was fortunate to have been born into a privileged family and stable economic society, circumstances that paved the way for me to achieve whatever I could.

As a child, life was understandable. Follow directions, work hard, care for one another, and the outcome was predictable. Society was orderly. For better or worse, people knew their places. Paternal authority was unquestioned, the police were our friends, and church was obligatory. As children we marched in parades on the Fourth of July and felt the pride of those who survived the two great wars in Europe.

The radio and newsprint of the day sheltered us from the graphic representations of human suffering. We were once shocked by the color images of starving Biafran children in *Life* magazine. The shock value wore off as Vietnam dragged on day after day and year after year. Televised scenes of human destruction and defoliation of the earth interrupted the peaceful family dinner.

The Vietnam War was too long and too close. People my age were serving, dying, or scarred for their lives. With educational deferments for most of the 1960s, I had time to wonder why. It was part of the student personality to resist and to question authority. The polarization of the 1960s forced a distinction between feeling good and doing good. Amid all the Chinese sloganeering, "Serve the people" remained as a clear goal for me. For many, it was a time to decide on the crossroads of life.

Early in my career, my clinical course was altered by several indelible medical experiences. While serving as a medical student on an exchange program in Karachi, Pakistan in the late 1960s, for example, I watched a child die as she waited in a protracted medical queue. When her turn came to be placed on the examination desk, doctors summarily discharged her distraught family. There was nothing left that they could do. In an instant I understood the life-saving role of public health and preventive medicine. Of course we can do more: cholera deaths can be prevented. It was an obvious decision. I would become a pediatrician with special training in public health and preventive medicine.

After medical school, internship, and 2 years as a general medical officer (GMO) in the U.S. Public Health Service, I was fortunate to receive a grant from the Robert Wood Johnson Foundation to study pediatrics, public health, and epidemiology at Johns Hopkins University. Over time as a general pediatrician, I was able to publish original research on tropical diseases such as onchocerciasis and domestic childhood injury problems such as poisonings and baby walker injuries. In addition, for a number of years I was able to produce an original public health radio broadcast on a local NBC station in central Massachusetts.

I have always been fascinated with adapting clinical care to people living in tribal society. During the 6 years between medical school and the completion of my pediatric residency and public health training, I worked as a clinician with the Cherokee and Shawnee tribes in Oklahoma and the Mandingo people in upcountry Liberia. I also worked as a researcher with the indigenous tribes of the Guatemalan highlands. These immersion experiences hit me over the head with cultural, linguistic, and traditional imperatives. Techniques learned in medical school took a back seat to the special nature of each person seated before me, and my key operatives became understanding, tolerance, and patience.

Looking back to my days as a recent graduate physician, I may have been overly eager to prove myself. I remember one experience as a fresh intern on rotation in the neonatal intensive care unit. I was called STAT to the nursery, and on my perceived rescue mission I actually unhinged a door that was ajar and difficult to open. Impressed with my earnest effort, the nursing staff decorated the doorway with an ornamental sign reading "Fazen's Folly." A year later, in northeast Oklahoma, I was a very young physician fresh from training in Chicago and Buffalo. Here, I received a blunt lesson about the inadvisability of rushing in before fully appreciating prevailing cultural norms. As a general medical officer for the Cherokee Nation, I possessed the necessary medical information, but my manner of delivery to the Cherokee elders was stiff and uncompromising. I knew what was medically indicated, but I overlooked the significance of the "Trail of Tears" and the proud Cherokee heritage *"Tsa-la-gi."* Although I worked long hours and had many positive patient interactions, one night I was called before the elders of the tribal council to explain my reluctance to prescribe simple antibiotics. I began to realize that effective physicians need to understand and serve communities as well as individuals.

While a student at Northwestern University Medical School 25 years ago, my professor, Dr. Y. Y. Hsia, suggested I might want to apply for a fellowship to work on diarrhea research in Pakistan. Either I wasn't much of an asset in the genetics lab or Dr. Hsia foresaw how the humanitarian mission would make a lasting impression on me. As I passed through Southeast Asia in 1968, I felt uniquely privileged to be an American male with a purpose unrelated to the war in Vietnam. Living with a Pakistani family, rounding at the Children's Hospital, and traveling throughout the country including the spectacular Himalayas, I came back a changed man and 35 pounds lighter. After their initial surprise, my parents also realized I would not be joining my father's surgical practice.

Since that time, I have worked as a salaried pediatrician in four different hospital systems. As a general pediatrician and a teacher, I have enjoyed a wide variety of clinical positions ranging from outpatient and critical care for pediatric inpatients to emergency medicine and now back to ambulatory medicine. Each hospital position involved the care of indigent populations, but my current position is the first to focus exclusively on the health problems of poverty since I worked for the Indian Health Service.

My resolve to take this position solidified recently, while I was living with my wife and three children in Africa for 1 year to teach at the University of Zimbabwe School of Medicine. While we were beginning to understand the ancient customs and traditions of the Shona people in that part of the world, the United States and its allies swarmed into Kuwait and then invaded Iraq. Discussions at the medical school centered around the neocolonial powers of the Northern Hemisphere and the oppression of the peoples of the South. In the end, the United States did not look victorious.

I was frequently faced with the dichotomy of CNN showing off our smart bombs of destruction while, at the same
time, the CDC was reporting outbreaks of measles in Houston
and Chicago. How could Zimbabwe have a better immunization rate for measles than the United States, one of the most
advanced nations in the world? Viewing our national priorities from afar led me to rearrange my own agenda. I decided
to combine clinical medicine and public health by accepting
a new position to direct a pediatrics program in Boston's inner city. Crisscrossing numerous roads, I found the way to
express my involvement with poor people of multiple cultural
and racial backgrounds and a Third-World heritage.

When I arrive at the clinic each day, I try to maintain
a sense of service as well as a sense of humor. I chuckle as
children and parents comment on my similarities to Mr. Rogers — his manners, appearance, and even voice. But this is
not Mr. Rogers' neighborhood. The headline today reads,
"President Clinton asks help on police sweeps in public housing." Reading the paper on the bus into town, I know what
we do is important because our unattended problems usually
surface as notorious casualties on the front page. In just over
an hour, as I travel from the suburbs into Boston's inner city,
many of life's problems do a flip-flop. Green becomes asphalt.
Being safe becomes providing security. Individual homes become apartments in high rise buildings.

The area outside the pediatric clinic window is a well-
lighted and airy space for children to play and parents to
wait. Today, the waiting room is filling up quickly; a 7-year-
old named Carlos is there with his mother and two siblings.
Sadie, our nursing assistant, calls for Carlos and begins the
necessary measurements before I can sit down with him. Carlos has headaches and behavioral problems in his second-
grade classroom. Further history reveals an abnormal sleep
pattern and major disciplinary problems at home.

Carlos' physical exam and neurological evaluation are
normal. It appears his headaches stem from a crowded and

turbulent home situation; meanwhile, his hyperactivity interferes with his school performance. We step out of the exam room to consider his case. Carlos was born into the village life of a Caribbean island culture. Uprooted with his mother and siblings, he landed in a disappointing and bewildering new world. Housing is in short supply, traditional family supports are lacking, and everyday life is complicated by confusing and often contradictory social values. We worry that this 7-year-old will not be able to adjust emotionally.

Carlos needs what each of us has to offer. Today there are just too many children born into poverty and too many families without health care and too many communities in turmoil with violence, drugs, and lack of education and jobs. During medical student education, residency training, and our professional careers, each of us is drawn more and more into the disturbing morass of caring for patients in the midst of social and economic disarray. Each day many health professionals across the country and around the world wrestle with the inequities of health.

Carlos will need a prescription medicine to reduce his hyperactivity, but it will take more to reduce the headaches. Do they have health insurance? There is a need to support home life, to improve community supports, and to provide psychological counseling. What about transportation? Do they have a phone? What resources does the school have? Where do we find a Spanish-speaking psychologist? Telephone calls and paper work ensue.

Last night a 15-year-old was shot in the face and neck on the basketball court just behind the Health Center. Everyone feels a heightened awareness of the fragility of life all around us. Was it the Academy Homes versus the Heath Street Boys settling some old scores? The shooting is not yet in the early morning paper, but our staff members, coffee in hand, are already trying to digest the news and sort out possible scenarios.

While scheduled patients are checked for temperature and weight, others are calling in for sick visits. The first patient is a 4-month-old taking prophylactic antibiotics for a kidney problem diagnosed *in utero*. Today his mother complains he is not eating well (the familiar "No quiere comida") and is "a little sad." What does it mean to be sad at 4 months of age? For assistance with translation I manage to pull Teresa away from her other duties. We learn his symptoms began 10 days ago, about the same time his father left home. When the mother starts crying in the exam room, Teresa's presence becomes particularly important; nursing human misery is a crucial step in easing disease, pain, and disability. The mother knows a psychologist at the Health Center and we facilitate her return visit. She departs with a *"muy amable"* (you are very kind) for each of us. As we walk out of the room, Teresa and I realize again why we are here. The "laying on of hands" provides more than diagnosis and treatment. The human touch transmits a sensation of hope for people in pain.

The lab tech calls with the results of Carlos' blood count. We plan to start Carlos on medication for hyperactivity and make an appointment to see him in 2 weeks to review his behavior and sleeping patterns. Down the hall in room 6, in the middle of the exam, a young patient can't hold back his curiosity. Even his family is surprised by his question: "Why is your nose too thin?" I never thought of it in those terms, but we all laugh as we compare noses in the exam room. Next is a boy with an old traumatic injury to his great toe. It is messy. He has not been seen, we are told, as his parents have recently separated. The child became an accessory, stranded in time between parents. He will need a dressing change and both parents to thrive.

Before I can see the next patient, Tata pulls me aside to explain the mother is *"muy preocupado."* She is very worried about a birthark on the abdomen of her newborn. Is it *"antajo?"* With Tata's help, I can understand the Dominican interpretation of a birth mark as a signal of the mother's cravings during pregnancy.

Maybe she had a craving for chocolate during gestation, as this benign nevus has a milk chocolate appearance. Moving on to the developmental assessment of an 18-month-old from a bilingual family, I inquire about his language skills. Oh, yes, his mother reports, he even calls to the dog. Well, does he use the English "dog" or the Spanish "*perro?*" "No, he shouts, 'Rascal.' "

In the next room, while checking a baby for a minor cold, I turn to see her mother asleep in the office chair. Reviewing the chart, I find the mother was considering a drug rehabilitation program at the last visit. Her child is still shortchanged. Still an infant, the child's scars of deprivation may not show up until a teacher writes back about problems in school. Trying to improve her mother's parenting skills now may be easier than working through her inevitable acting-out behaviors in 15 years. We hope our social worker can spend some time with her mother to review the options to stop "using it."

Down the hall is a 4-year-old with wax in his ears complaining of "ninja turtles in there." The mother of a 1-year-old with recurrent pneumonia has returned. We had to discuss the blood test for AIDS. She probably suspected this possibility, but she was acutely distressed just the same. Then Dr. Joe, my colleague, calls me to the exam room to describe a rare case of "Norwegian" scabies in a tiny Latino infant. There is more to learn each day.

These are the problems of impoverished people. These are also the problems of society at large. In fact, divorce, drug addiction, domestic violence, and street crimes occur in all strata of society and in all our neighborhoods. In the inner city, the accompanying problems of low income, poor insurance, insufficient education with high illiteracy, and little hope of altering the situation leave people particularly devastated. A drug-addicted person with adequate resources — family and supportive community, health insurance, financial reserves and education — can usually navigate out of a difficult situation. In poverty, the added problems become cumulative, and it appears impossible to dig out.

Finally, Sadie and I are able to take a few minutes to review Carlos' history. His teacher called because she was worried about his classroom behavior and thought it important to investigate the headaches. She has requested a physical exam and involvement in the home by the state Department of Social Services. His mother lives alone with Carlos and two other siblings: an older sister, Emelita, and a 2-year-old brother, Juan. She is not mean spirited, but she is plainly overwhelmed. She frequently confronts Carlos, trying to get him to calm down, especially at 4 in the morning, when he awakens and disturbs the household. Underneath all his disorderly conduct, Carlos is a very unhappy little boy. Lacking a father presence and any sufficient coping mechanisms, given his level of stress, he is acting out his fantasies of isolation, remorse, and lost hopes.

We understand his frustrations are climbing to the boiling point. Sadie wonders if it would be possible to arrange for a male teacher or a Big Brothers program before it is too late? We need more time to make calls and check on funding and determine transportation in the event community resources can be found for him. And time is running out.

I was prepared for this work by some influential mentors. Certainly, my wife has been my most steadfast supporter through all the years. A special person with an innate sense of grace, she provides the "crazy glue" of good humor and common sense essential to a happy family environment. A physician with advanced training in pediatrics, Lynn Eckhert also holds a doctorate degree in Maternal and Child Health from Johns Hopkins University. As a mother of three energetic children, a wife, and a distinguished physician and administrator, Lynn seems to thrive with many irons in the fire at one time. Although she travels frequently throughout the country and at times around the world, she is always just a phone call away. After 25 years of marriage, we still endeavor to make each other laugh at least once a day.

Lynn is adept at recognizing the difference between sharing a profession and raising a family together, and the need for each of us to find our own career pathways. We each understand and appreciate the work of the other, but at the same time we thrive on the individuality associated with separate workplaces. To enable full pursuit of our professional lives, we fortunately found loving and capable providers during our children's younger years.

In a strict sense, I never had the kind of mentor one could follow up the traditional ladder of achievement. My attempt to combine international health experiences with ongoing primary care in the American community is not a typical medical model. This combination has been done before, but it is an uncharted course with uncertain endpoints. Without a mentor for credibility, some of my actions and problem-solving approaches have at times been considered strange by my peers and direct supervisors. Once I was called in by my director to explain why I appear to question authority. Actually I prefer not so much to question authority but, as my bumper sticker reads, to "Question Reality." In the end I seem to be appreciated much more by the staff who work directly with me than by my supervisors. The person-to-person recognition has been my most consistent reward for the work I do.

My mentors, then, did not hold my career advancement in their grasp but rather offered inspiration from a distance. I have known a number of outstanding individuals who were simply doing what they considered important regardless of the changing winds of economics, politics, or the prevailing medical thought. International Health Professors Carl Taylor and Tim Baker at Johns Hopkins University, for example, are people woven from a unique cloth. They have been able to combine medical wisdom, the health needs of large populations, and love of people into their teaching careers in public health. In addition, I turn to doctors Hugh Fulmer, an early and ardent spokesperson for community-oriented primary care, and Leonard Morse, a natural-born leader in Worcester medicine and president of the Massachusetts Medical Society. Finally, over the past decade, our minister, Mike Scrogin, has preached the connectedness of people, the value of community, and the spiritual basis of existence: the necessary tendons holding life together. These people provided inspiration over the years when iconoclastic approaches to health care were on the wane.

My wife and I are unified in our love for medical and health care projects overseas. During our travels, many people around the world helped to shape our personal beliefs and our sense of a shared world existence. Experiences on three continents have rewarded my wife and me with an invigorated sense of purpose in our personal lives and professional careers. Back home I like to conjure up images of the global village we have visited over the past 25 years. My wife and I have assembled a photographic exhibit of faces and places in Africa, Asia, and Latin America where we have learned and helped in some small way. The color images of our global family represent people and places in and around our medical work sites in the developing world.

Many of the photographs were taken in the days before the airbus and satellite communication and the worldwide effects of merging, shrinking, and commercializing life-styles. In the early days after medical school and public health training, the landing of a Boeing 707 in Karachi or Kabul was an event of wonderment, as early technology brought the unknown to the inaccessible. Twenty-five years ago tribal life dominated the landscape more than superpower detente. A multitude of distant, discrepant villages seemed to preclude the concept of the global family.

"Code Gray! Code Gray!" Today the whole place smelled of bleach. Strong bleach; 100% bleach. Two women in the pediatric waiting room got into a terrible ruckus and in the end became violent. In response to the "Code Gray" I arrived to find myself in the thick of it. No one was seriously injured, but the blood had to be cleaned up, and onlooking patients and their children needed reassurance. It is personally insulting to be physically wounded by another person. It demeans our existence together. Last year I was hit in the face with a mace solution from a spray bottle outside the health center. Initially I felt victimized. Later, with support from staff and friends, I found serenity believing my work in some way might eventually reduce the anger leading to random violence.

There is a great opportunity here for me to use my best clinical skills to help others in need and then to pass along some of that end-of-the-day excitement to other health center staff, students, and residents in training as well as to my own family. Unfortunately, it doesn't always work that way. First of all, our health care delivery system is difficult to synchronize with our patient's needs. Although the patients present a delightful array of colorful personalities, and our staff does a remarkable job of working together despite our differences in culture, race, and economic status, we often end the day with headaches of frustration.

Many of our patients do not fit into mainstream medical systems. They dwell in the slipstream of society. We seem to be chronically underfunded to do what is medically necessary for them as well as what the patients want us to do and the malpractice lawyers expect us to do. For more than 3 years we have wondered about ways to be more accessible to our patients with evening hours and weekend care, but somehow the solution has eluded us. Many of our patients do not come as scheduled each day. In addition, we are funded to do categorical projects but are often unable to fully integrate these special projects with our daily medical care. We utilize difficult computer systems that are unfriendly to both providers and patients. The talented staff, the basic resources, and the needy patients are all here, but somehow it becomes cumber-

some and stressful for us to serve our community. I know we
are doing the right thing, but I wish it felt better, better for
all of us.

However, each day in the red brick health center brings
fascinating insight into the extravagant dilemmas existing
within urban poverty. After all, we are of a very rich country
with a long tradition of democratic ideals, and yet neither
the market economy nor the political will serves the best interests of the patients we see each day. Maybe there is a
crossroad for people from all backgrounds to fulfill our prom-
ises from the original Bill of Rights to President Johnson's
pronouncement on the Great Society and the War on Poverty.
We have a stake in human equity and a need to promote
basic living communities and a chance for individual happiness. Each life fulfills a purpose. In Zimbabwe, "*Musha
Mukadzi*" is the Shona tribal custom of embellishing the family home to promote the well-being of the extended family,
the tribe, and the wide community surrounding us. As an
African aphorism holds, it takes a whole village to raise a
single child.

In her role as a nursing assistant, Sadie has been helping
families almost since the center opened 28 years ago. Sadie
is only one of many health professionals at all levels who for
generations have migrated to mission posts around the world
and to concentrations of people in need in this country in
health centers like ours. At Carlos' age Sadie was picking cotton. She grew up in a large family in a small home in rural
Alabama. As a teen-ager she migrated away from her family
with the hope of a better life in the North. Forty years later,
she continues on with the compassion and charm of someone
who knows the value of each day. Sadie defines the grace we
are looking for in our daily lives.

And all our patients pass our sentinel, Manny, at the
door. Manny is a broad black man from western Africa. He
is firm with those who need to find their place and taciturn
with his everyday customers. You don't go to Manny with idle

conversation, but just ask him to sing. He has a resonant baritone honed on African church music. Manny adds the texture to our Christmas sing and our Martin Luther King Day celebrations. Just imagine Manny as the anchor with our health center staff singing the traditional Negro spiritual: *Live a-Humble:*

Live a hum-ble, ____ humble, ____ Humble your-selves,
  the bells's done rung.
Glo-ry and hon-or! ____ Glo-ry and hon-or! ____

Praise King Je-sus! Praise the Lord!
Live a hum-ble, ____ humble, ____ Humble your-selves,
  the bells's done rung.

I want to acknowledge the cadre of dedicated support staff, nurses, and physicians who have concentrated their whole lives on the problems of providing health care for needy people. In each community we know who they are.

Last week I had a chance to visit Carlos in his classroom. In my presence he behaved as a perfect gentleman. He spontaneously wrote in English for the first time ever, and his teacher couldn't believe her eyes. He obviously responds to the supportive adult male role. It is amazing to consider this male coming from a foreign culture and language and from the other end of the social, economic, and educational scale could provide the necessary calming influence. Carlos gave me a real hug at the end of class. I was privileged to be there for him.

The Maternal and Infant Care Committee meets monthly, a gathering of dedicated health center providers in multiple areas to meet to discuss relevant issues. The committee of 20 or so are almost all women, experienced caregivers with children of their own. Health risks during pregnancy can be divided into medical and social areas. The purely medical risks are nearly the same for any woman from any part of society; unfortunately, here, the social issues predominate. Is the mother herself a child? How did she become pregnant? Was it a forced or loving relationship? Is there a possibility of a sexually transmitted disease? And the list goes on to include safety issues, substance abuse, housing, the role of the father, questions about terminating the pregnancy, family support, schooling, transportation, telephone, and compliance with medical recommendations. We spend precious time discussing options for the socially disordered: evasive mothers who just refuse to address their addictions and chaotic life-style even if it affects the unborn.

From my own experience, I know the difficulty of making good decisions on family issues, even with years of parenting behind me, medical expertise, and financial resources. Often, I reflect on the common needs of all children as well as the universal pressures on parents trying to do the best they can with what they have. This caring committee is full of the technical expertise and the human compassion necessary to improve maternal and child health, but we don't have safe homes with good food and a consistent, loving family to offer. Those are the gems of existence. From our caseload, we know what it means to try to get by without the essentials in life.

The refrigerator in pediatrics is chock full of home-cooked specialties. Sadie, Tata, and Teresa and I have each made a favorite dish. Today we have another going-away party. This is a special time of wonderful food and companionship made bittersweet by the sad news that another valued member of the staff is departing. It takes a long time to learn the ways of the professional life of the health center. Standard diagnoses and treatments are just the beginning; we need to know all the other variables affecting health care for people with inadequate resources. Just following the names of family members — immediate and extended — and their relations to other families is very complex. Are they still living in Boston, or have they returned to the Dominican Republic? Sorting through these social issues begins anew with the orientation of each recent employee.

The food is colorful and plentiful. We enjoy some favorite home recipes as the staff takes pride in serving others. We gather in random groupings distinct from our working teams, and I hear about the concerns of another department. There is laughter as we recount goings-on in the neighborhood. We are happy as a family can be. Our racial, ethnic, and cultural differences only serve to spice up the occasion. There is a special bond of sharing a meal together, the communal aspect of breaking bread. Thoughtful gifts reflect a natural outpouring of human kindness and genuine concern for others. Some of the presents come from the tradition of another world in Latin America. The *"sombrilla"* or decorative parasol with confetti always seems to surprise the expectant mother at her baby shower. Another gift is much appreciated — the envelope with a cash donation. There is wishing well all around.

The phones are ringing, and it's back to work. Carlos had to be hospitalized for threatening behaviors. This will bring in a new set of caregivers, new ideas, and new medications. His story is not going to resolve very soon. This kind of healing takes a long time. And we continue on, together.

POSTSCRIPT

Dr. Louis Fazen recently left his position at the Martha Elliot Health Center. Following a vacation in Argentina, he will seek another position in Boston serving disadvantaged populations. At present, Dr. Fazen is submitting his *Expanded Program for Immunization* for publication. He is also serving as a consultant for both the Maryland State Department of Health and The Johns Hopkins School of Hygiene and Public Health's Preventive Medicine Residency.

CHAPTER V

A VOICE FOR THE PUBLIC'S HEALTH

DONALD P. FRANCIS, M.D., D.SC.

There was no hesitation in my voice. There was no hesitation in my body language. I was on course, the right course. But what I was saying was not pleasant. I was criticizing the actions of my honored and revered Centers for Disease Control (CDC), and I was criticizing the President of the United States. I spoke the truth about how America's public health had been jeopardized by the Reagan and Bush Administrations. I described how the CDC was prevented from doing its job by political extremism and a loss of understanding of the federal government's responsibility for epidemic control. It was June 1992, the 21st anniversary of my public health career.

Sitting at the Capitol Hill witness table with Bud Roper, who directed the Roper opinion polls, I looked up at Congressman Ted Weiss, the subcommittee chairman. He listened intently to Mr. Roper's and my testimony. He listened as Mr. Roper described the results of his recent poll, which showed that Americans felt personally threatened by the AIDS epidemic and were ready for frank and forthright messages on how to prevent sexual and drug-use-associated HIV infection. He listened intently as I, a career officer of the Centers for Disease Control, described how the previous Reagan Administration and the present Bush Administration had successfully prevented the launching of an HIV prevention program worthy of the dangers posed by that virus. In my 10-minute testimony I impugned the very government public health institutions that I had represented in epidemic control programs around the world.

Why me? Why was I destined to sit before a Congressional committee to berate a powerful administration for public health malpractice?

The reasons can perhaps be traced back to the 1950s westerns that I watched on our family's first television. The white-hatted cowboys on *Bar 7 Theater* never backed down from what was right, even if it hurt them. These shows, through a cloud of macho naiveté with their good-guys-always-win theatrics, instilled an impression that the good guy rather than the brute will be victorious eventually. Today that naiveté still exists in me, modified somewhat by the realities of life's experience, which have taught me that, at least in the short run, brutes often do quite well.

But the *Bar 7 Theater* cannot take all the credit. My ability to stand strong and often alone against adversity has its roots with my parents. At dinner one night in our comfortable house in Marin County, California, I made a joke about Arkansas Governor Orville Faubus' attempt to maintain segregation of blacks. In 1959, the federal government was taking on states like Arkansas that wanted to maintain the "separate-but-equal" stance of the segregationists. Governor Faubus had made a national plea to send him money so he and his white supremacists could withstand the force of the federal authorities. In cynical jest, I suggested that we all send him money — Confederate money. My parents laughed at the joke but wouldn't let it drop. My father suggested I call Herb Caen, a columnist with the *San Francisco Chronicle* and tell him about my idea. At lunch break the next day, I went to the telephone booth in front of the gymnasium at Redwood High School and called him with my idea. That Sunday, my plea to send Confederate money to the segregationists was the lead paragraph in his column, and soon I was on the front page of papers around the country. Considering the value of true Confederate dollars, I adjusted my plea to send imitation Confederate bills — and they arrived by the pound.

My parents were both doctors — my mother a radiologist, my father an internist. My grandfather on my father's side was also a doctor. But my interest in medicine was not stimulated actively by my parents. In a way, their realization of the consuming training and the chaotic life of a physician seemed at times to have discouraged my parents from directing me toward medicine. This was especially true for my mother. She was a beautiful and brilliant woman, in Stanford at the age of 15 years and one of the first female radiologists trained in their program. She, like most women doctors, was always torn between her career in medicine and her obligation to her children. She did a great balancing job. She would go to her office in San Rafael in the morning and come home to read her X-rays in the afternoon.

In a most subtle way, she was always protective of her boys, wanting the best, yet letting them learn for themselves. I can recall that she strongly imposed her will only a few times. On one notable occasion, it had to do with our vocabulary. We were raised in a permissive home with little censoring of our cursing, but Beth wouldn't tolerate one word: "nigger." I remember bringing it home from school as a derogatory term that I didn't understand but still used without hesitation. For the first time, I saw the hair raise on her neck and, in a very clear voice, she asked if I knew what it meant. I didn't and admitted it.

She explained it and, in her simple but straightforward way, stated that with our long family associations in Texas and Arizona, it would not be surprising if we had black relatives. "Would you like to be called a nigger?" she asked. I never used it again. Recently, I had the same discussion with my boys about "homo" and "queer."

Despite her strong feelings, she rarely tried to influence my brother's or my own important life decisions. I do, however, recall how she reacted when I announced that I was going to become a pediatrician. She strongly objected, fearing that my home life would be destroyed by patient obligations. She was similarly protective about my work in the tropics. She, being wiser than I, recognized the risks I exposed myself to by working with infectious diseases in inherently dangerous parts of the world. Her "be careful" admonitions when I would announce another even more dangerous assignment were greeted by me in a similar way to when I was a teenager and she cautioned me about driving. Little did I know how much she knew and how important her advice was on both counts. However, I ignored most of it, and she allowed it.

My father was even more reserved and just plain supportive of whatever decision Steve, my brother, or I would make. Indeed, getting advice from him was very difficult. He came from an English family in which emotions were buried far below the surface. When major issues emerged, his reluctantly offered advice was immensely valuable. My father, Cy, although trained in internal medicine, became a high-level administrator in the Veterans Administration. Drafted from a Beverly Hills medical practice into the Navy during World War II, he not so accurately predicted that socialized or centralized medicine would imminently come to the United States. Considering this prediction — perhaps 50 years too early — he wanted to be in on the ground floor of its organization. He believed that the Veterans Administration (VA) would be the cutting edge of universal health care, and he wanted to be there. Over the years, he became increasingly frustrated with the VA's bureaucracy and disillusioned with our government's ability to function. When I began my government career and confronted bureaucratic obstacles, his advice to me was, "Don, as an administrator, you have to constantly walk on the edge of being fired. If you want to accomplish any positive change, you will have to take risks." If he had only lived long enough to see his son repeat his administrative style.

As time went on, my parents' support allowed me to successfully negotiate the multiple crises of the 1960s. The major crisis was the war. It was the Vietnam War that really brought forth courage in all of us who confronted the establishment and opposed that disgraceful national action. We were forced to stand alone, different, and often despised. In 1968, I began medical school at Northwestern University in Chicago. Dr. Seifert, a semiretired physician who directed the University Health Clinic, inspired my interest in infectious diseases by describing such tropical diseases as diphtheria, polio, tetanus, and measles. Although fascinated, I found that concentrating exclusively on my medical career ignored a far greater injustice inflicted on the poor villagers of Southeast Asia not by tropical diseases but by our bombers. I helped found a chapter of activist health science students called the Student Health Organization (SHO). We staffed a free clinic on the western side of Chicago, organized antiwar protests, and counseled draft evaders.

Although a number of medical students at Northwestern shared my social concerns, many more were mostly concerned, over and above studying for exams, with memorizing sports trivia or investing in the stock market. I addressed a letter to them as I approached my last days in Chicago. I urged them to become involved with the impoverished members of our society and to resist the draft.

Confronted with a medical student writing such a letter, the dean asked me to come to his office. I had been wanting to talk to him anyway because I had received an international pediatric fellowship in India for my last quarter of medical school and was going to ask if I could be excused from graduation ceremonies. But after my appointment, I never had to ask.

From the moment I entered his office he castigated me for my stance against the war. He screamed at the top of his lungs across his huge hardwood desk, "You are a disgrace to the medical profession!" At first I tried to explain my reasoning, that I wasn't really so disgraceful. But he was out of control and beyond any attempt at reason. At the conclusion of his diatribe, he ordered me not to come to the graduation. During the shouting I was scared. It was far from pleasant, being chastised by the pinnacle of the medical school administration. Strangely, although I felt very uncomfortable with the situation, I felt comfortable with my position. And, as time passed, I felt proud that I withstood such a lonely and brutal attack with honor and poise — far more, indeed, than that shown by the not-so-fine dean.

I learned from my faculty contacts that the dean had petitioned the faculty committee to officially chastise or possibly expel me. He presented my letter to the faculty and asked for comments from the chair of psychiatry, who, after reading the letter, commented, "It's one of the best things I've read." With that, the dean's balloon collapsed, and months later I received a diploma in the mail.

Our antiwar protests in Chicago culminated with the 1968 Democratic convention. Months spent planning for demonstrations ultimately resulted in a barbaric police attack, which showed the American public how brutish our government had become. Fortunately for my scalp, by the time of the convention I was in India, pursuing my professional interest in infectious diseases — this time controlling tetanus of the newborn at the foot of the Himalayas.

When I came back to the United States in January 1969, the ferment over the war was continuing, and I returned to the fray. By then I was a doctor. Indeed, I was a third-

generation California physician, beginning a pediatric internship at Los Angeles County/USC Medical Center, the very
place where my father had been an intern 30 years before.

At that time in American history, young doctors were
clearly rocking the boat. Each month we held "Moratorium
Days" during which we lined tables in the hallways of the
hospital with literature and anti-war buttons. Speakers were
invited to the center of the hospital grounds to address the
atrocities of the war and the lies peddled by our government.
On special days, marches consisting of thousands of protesters crossed Los Angeles.

We defined medical responsibility differently than in the
past. Maintaining the status quo as supported by the more
conservative practitioners of medicine was no longer acceptable. Many older physicians confronted us about our stands,
our clothes, and our hair. There was constant pressure to con-
form and no pleasure in these confrontations. Each one made
me uncomfortable because many came from doctors who were
my mentors; I respected them for their expertise and appreciated their medical teachings. What helped me most to withstand this pressure were the few supporters within "the
system" who, although they may not have agreed with our
tactics, supported our right to speak and appreciated our expressions of social concern.

As my parents had done earlier in my life, it was supportive people like these who granted me the strength to
carry on, to fight, and to follow my chosen path. These few
sentinel people have guided me and given me courage
throughout my training and career. I am forever indebted to
them. The first of these experiences occurred during my first
year of medical school. It was a miserable year, and I yearned
to do something more relevant and pleasurable. During the
following summer, I visited Roger Nichols, a professor of mine
at Berkeley in whose laboratory I had worked during my last
two years at Cal. I told him I wanted to quit medical school
and return to Berkeley to pursue a doctorate in medical phys-

ics. He, together with Dr. John Lawrence of the Donnor Laboratory, sat me down and explained why it was worthwhile to put up with the misery and complete medical school. In clear terms, they showed me how much better it would be for me to get my M.D. and, only later, return for my Ph.D. That hour changed my whole life, for it was medicine that has been central to my professional and political accomplishments. Later, I did get a doctorate in virology from Harvard, but even this work was focused on preventing infectious diseases in people.

At the conclusion of my second year of pediatric training in Los Angeles, I received another round of critical guidance and advice. With over 95% of doctors being drafted, it became increasingly clear that my conscientious objector application would be rejected by my draft board and I would be required to enter the military and support the Vietnam War. Being adamantly against the war, yet not wanting to go to jail, I decided to move to Canada. I made an appointment with Dr. Paul Wehrle, the chief of pediatrics at LAC/USC Medical Center, to get his advice about a good hospital in Canada where I could finish my pediatric and infectious disease training. Paul had been one of those supporters who, regardless of how clumsily I had protested some social inadequacy, always understood my goals. He counseled me on better ways to achieve them rather than lecturing me on the disturbance I had caused.

At this meeting, Paul asked, "Why don't you apply for the EIS program at CDC in Atlanta?" I knew about the Centers for Disease Control in Atlanta but had never heard of the Epidemic Intelligence Service (EIS). He explained that 2 years chasing epidemics would qualify for military duty, and, should I be accepted, I would not have to move to Canada. I enlisted for 2 years and stayed for over 20.

The CDC was just the spot for me. I was very interested in pediatric infectious disease, but, unknown to me, I had become increasingly interested in preventive medicine and public health. In infectious disease the first case of an unusual disease is always a wonderful experience. I will never forget my first cases of tetanus, meningitis, whooping cough, diphtheria, malaria, botulism, tuberculosis, and typhoid fever.

But treating some of these diseases can be extremely difficult. I remember most notably baby boy Stills, a young poor child from central Los Angeles with whooping cough. Every night, just after dinner, he would have such severe coughing that he would have a cardiac arrest. We would all rush to his bedside and spend hours reviving him. My interest in this fascinating disease subsided as the grueling need to care for him became routine. Baby boy Stills lived, but not without extensive costs and misery to him, his family, and the hospital staff who cared for him. And it was all preventable. Baby boy Stills had not received his baby shots. One of these, the "P" of DPT, would have completely prevented the entire 6-week episode. I pledged to myself that all babies under my care would be immunized. Never should a preventable disease be allowed to torture such young and innocent victims. Unknown to me, that was one of the principal roles of CDC.

My first assignment was to the State Health Department in Portland, Oregon. Before I even found a house, I found myself in eastern Oregon battling an outbreak of bubonic plague. In the year and a half I stayed in Oregon, I fought outbreaks of measles, diphtheria, hepatitis, and leptospirosis. But the finale was the smallpox outbreak that was imported into Yugoslavia. With only 2 hours' notice I was asked to pack my bags and join a team of about ten CDC people in Washington, D.C. for immediate departure to Yugoslavia. A pilgrim to Mecca had traveled through Iraq on his return and imported smallpox to the southern, largely Muslim area of Yugoslavia. Within weeks, combined American and Yugoslavian teams stopped the outbreak with aggressive vaccination. Without that effort, it would have spread throughout the country and beyond.

Following the Yugoslavian smallpox outbreak, I met perhaps my most influential guideperson, Bill Foege. After defeating smallpox in Yugoslavia in 1972, I met Bill at a smallpox division picnic in Atlanta en route to Portland. Unfortunately for me, I met him first on the opposite side of a volleyball net. Bill, being 6 foot 7 inches, is not the person to face in volleyball. He had no mercy and pummeled me with spikes and lobs.

Still dripping with sweat caused by the combination of volleyball and the intense tropical air of Atlanta, I told him that I enjoyed beating back smallpox in Yugoslavia and that, if he ever planned a larger effort and needed help, I would join. A few months later, the CDC, World Health Organization, and several other countries began "Target Zero," the worldwide campaign that 5 years later eliminated smallpox from the world. I first went to Sudan, where I headed the national program. Sudan, the largest country in Africa, had only 250 miles of paved roads. I spent the better part of a year in a Land Rover covering all corners of the country, searching for cases of smallpox. Sudan, extending from the southern edge of the Sahara to the northern edge of tropical central Africa, is a wonderful country. I found excellent people working in the most difficult conditions. They eradicated smallpox despite the absence of roads, hotels, cafes, or telephones. They did it well, and they did it with honor. I watched them work with northern Arabs who had swords hanging at their waists and with southern blacks who had stretched earlobes and ivory bracelets.

The Sudan should be a prosperous country. It has a well-educated elite, great natural resources, and a cultural quality of honesty and integrity seldom seen elsewhere. After smallpox, I returned to Sudan twice, once for an outbreak of Ebola virus in 1976 and once 9 years later to help them with AIDS. On both return visits, the quality of life had noticeably decreased — and it had started low. The Arabs have been fighting against the southern blacks; the Muslims were fighting against the non-Muslims. And the economy, the pride and the honor of the country declined, all because of a few brutes whose selfish desire for power drove an already impoverished and abused people to a worse state.

After Sudan, WHO transferred me to India for "the big one." The major concentration of smallpox left in the world was on the Indian subcontinent. Bill Foege, my boss and my inspiration, had come to India with his family. It was a hard, often uncomfortable, and frustrating battle. We were naive thinking that several of us with a few extra vehicles could wipe out a scourge that had been consuming parts of a whole continent for a century. We started by recruiting all health workers for 1 week to search all villages for any evidence of smallpox. Bill Foege had discovered when he was working on smallpox eradication in Nigeria that by searching out every single outbreak and vaccinating everyone in contact with each case, smallpox could be controlled and, because there was no animal host for the virus, eliminated.

After months of frustration in India, we regrouped, got additional resources from the Swedish government, and launched a major attack in the wet and muddy monsoon season, when the virus transmission was lower. Soon cases began to drop, and a few months later there was no case to be found.

I had to cut short my assignment in India when my mother was diagnosed with nasopharyngeal carcinoma. I went home to comfort her and get her stabilized, but I returned to the subcontinent for a few months to help out a troubled program in Bangladesh. Again I was fortunate to see smallpox go from a pancountry epidemic, killing, blinding, and scarring people by the thousands, to a disease only in the history books. The exhilaration of beating back such a horrible disease rests with each of us who took part in the eradication program. Few other experiences in life could be as fulfilling as being part of history's first successful eradication program.

The ideas and the execution of such an effort are the result of a few people who cared enough to take it on. Bill Foege was the catalyst. He later became the director of CDC and now, as the Executive Director of the Carter Presidential Center, continues to be a great inspiration to everyone who is trying to make the world a better place.

Having been "in the bush" for so long, I felt scientifically behind and desired to be reeducated on my return. Fortunately, CDC granted my request of support for additional training. I had initially planned to undertake a fellowship in infectious disease and study for a Masters in Public Health but felt that the M.P.H. was too general and somewhat duplicative of what I had already learned in the field. After discussing my plans with several people at CDC, I decided to combine my infectious disease fellowship with laboratory research in virology. With the help of Alex Langmuir, the former head of epidemiology at CDC and then professor at Harvard, I found Max Essex, a virologist studying feline leukemia virus (FeLV). As I had become increasingly interested in the late manifestations of viral infections, feline leukemia was an ideal bug to study. Unlike acute infections such as chickenpox, the common cold, or influenza, which induce disease within days of infection, viruses like FeLV don't show up for months to years after infection.

Ultimately, I spent 3 years at Harvard studying the transmission and natural history of FeLV. During that time, I gained immense respect for that virus, which, without outward signs of infection, would slowly destroy the immune system of cats, leading to cancer or opportunistic infections. Without knowing it, I was being incredibly well prepared for my work on AIDS, which, still hidden, had already been introduced into the United States. Simultaneously, I was awarded a doctorate in virology by Harvard.

But, at the time, there were no virus infections of humans that fit the model of FeLV, and I needed to find a good assignment with CDC to continue my career. The closest match was with the Hepatitis Division in Phoenix, Arizona. Hepatitis B virus, although not producing immunologic disease, did produce chronic hepatitis, cirrhosis, and cancer of the liver — sometimes decades after initial infection. The match was excellent, not only with my interest and experience with slow viruses but also with my interest in vaccines. Merck and Company was developing a new vaccine for hepatitis B virus, and my challenge was to test its effectiveness.

Testing the hepatitis B vaccine filled in the final piece of experience necessary to prepare me for the AIDS epidemic — working with gay men. As the highest-risk group for hepatitis B infection in the United States, gay men were an ideal group in which to study the effects of a preventive vaccine. Toward the end of my study of the vaccine's efficacy in 1981, Jim Curran, an epidemiologist in Atlanta working in sexually transmitted diseases, called to tell me about a new disease in gay men that caused immunosuppression and cancer.

Before long, I was asked by CDC to move to Atlanta to head up CDC's laboratory efforts to find the cause of AIDS, which we presumed was infectious. I naively accepted the challenge without knowing the impossibility of the assignment. From what the newly elected Reagan administration had done to my plans to eliminate hepatitis B infection in the United States, I knew that the financial commitment to disease prevention was limited, but I thought that a new epidemic like AIDS would not be ignored, even by the most conservative ideologue. Little did I know what was in store. I was asked to establish a laboratory to discover the cause of AIDS without enough money to buy equipment, to travel to get patient specimens, or to hire staff. Collaboration with others was the only way to accomplish my goal, and I started with Max Essex, my mentor at Harvard. Max worked closely with Bob Gallo at Harvard, and I, ultimately, with the Institut Pasteur in Paris. I supplied specimens from a variety of CDC studies to all of them to help them in their work and followed all leads in our limited lab at CDC. Eventually the

Institut Pasteur identified the virus, and we worked with them to prove that it caused the disease. But, working in parallel at the National Cancer Institute, Bob Gallo was given credit for the discovery. I was caught in the middle as an American government scientist trying to defend French scientists against the claims by another American government scientist.

In the face of absent commitment by the Reagan Administration to do anything about AIDS and the unpleasant relationships between CDC and NCI, I increasingly directed my efforts at prevention of AIDS. I was asked by CDC to design a national prevention program. Plans for that program were sent to Washington for funding. They were returned without support. At that point, I was caught between a well-trained responsibility to prevent disease and a higher administrative authority telling me to do nothing. I then asked CDC to send me to California. California was not only my home, but was also a place where action on HIV prevention was already gaining steam. I spent the next 7 years helping design prevention programs that now serve as models for much of the rest of the world.

But my troubles with Washington followed me to California, and I had to ask for help from the good people who had already done so much for me. Bill Foege and Jonas Salk (with whom I began working on an AIDS vaccine after arriving in California) joined together to help me through perhaps my greatest crisis, the attempt by the U.S. Government to fire me from CDC. The crisis centered around the publication of Randy Shilts' book *And the Band Played On.* I served as one of many sources of information for that book, which reviewed the inadequacies of the early responses to AIDS. It was critical of the Reagan Administration for their lack of leadership, of the blood banks for their ostrich approach to preventing transfusion-associated AIDS, and of Dr. Robert Gallo of the National Institutes of Health. When the book was published, my critical comments were clearly reported, especially through my official memos, which I had given to Shilts. A few weeks later, I was asked to come to Atlanta to meet "regarding my future career plans."

In California we had organized a coalition of physicians, public health workers, and other AIDS-concerned groups. This coalition was making progress toward designing and delivering an effective AIDS prevention program. With such progress, I was happy with the job and had asked CDC to extend the assignment for 4 years, at which time I could retire from the Public Health Service.

Washington had different ideas. On the days prior to my visit to Atlanta, they had ordered CDC to fire me. I learned the specifics of this order much later. What confronted me at the time was the smiling face of Dr. Jim Mason, then the Director of CDC, as he reached over his wide table in his office and said, "Don, I'm glad you will be coming back to Atlanta to work on tuberculosis." Stunned at being transferred from my post in California to Atlanta to work on a bacterial disease, I said little to Dr. Mason. Later, talking to Walt Dowdle, Mason's deputy, I learned that the transfer had nothing to do with my performance or CDC's desires. "It's all ordered by Washington." he explained.

Angered by the repression and tempted to respond forcefully, I sought guidance from Bill Foege and Jonas Salk. They both advised me against any aggressive retort. Instead, they both assured me that they would work with CDC to assign me either to the Carter Presidential Center or the Salk Institute to continue my work in California. They helped me write a diplomatic letter to Jim Mason that explained why my work in California was important and why it was well suited to me and valuable to CDC and the nation. Among other things, the letter pointed out that CDC had sent me to Harvard for a doctorate in retrovirology rather than tuberculosis and that working with AIDS was, therefore, far better suited to my expertise. The letter was proper and respectful; yet, with the help of Bill and Jonas, it carried a strong punch. It made CDC look inappropriate if they sent me back to Atlanta for tuberculosis.

Jim Mason immediately recognized the power of the letter. I was told he was furious and said that I had written the letter for the press. At that point, the press knew nothing about the letter. However, they were on the trail. By the time I returned to California from Atlanta, the television show *60 Minutes* called to asked if I was being punished for expressing my opinions. I told them that my assignment was being reviewed "as a routine," and I didn't think there would be any problems. But I knew, and Jim Mason knew, that if they tried to punish me, the press would come down on CDC unmercifully. The book had cast me as somewhat of a hero within the bureaucracy, and the press would have loved to confront CDC on my behalf. In addition, Art Agnos, the Mayor of San Francisco, in whose office I worked one day a week, had assured me that he would join with Foege and Salk to defend me against any adversity. He was the chair of the AIDS Committee of the U.S. Conference of Mayors and carried substantial weight. Fortunately, CDC recognized their situation and repulsed the attack from Washington. Mason left me in California, and I quietly retired in February 1992.

Now, I've merged my past experiences of vaccines and AIDS to try to develop an HIV vaccine. I have joined Genentech, a biotech company in South San Francisco, where much of the most advanced AIDS vaccine work has taken place. In my spare time, I am working with an international group of concerned persons to establish a large fund to ensure that advances in AIDS vaccine development can be made available to the world's developing countries.

I don't want to give the impression that help from the important people in my life was always associated with some cataclysmic career decision or that it always came from big name leaders. In the most disparate and distant lands in which I have worked, I have had the fortune of being helped by people constituted of gold. In Nigeria, it was Patrick

Gbarara; in Sudan, Abdel Gadir and Dr. Omer el Haj; in India, Rajinder Singh and Dr. M. I. D. Sharma; and in China, Dr. Xu Zhi-yi. I miss them all. If I could, I would have them around me no matter what I was doing. It is with them that the credit belongs for such great accomplishments as eradicating smallpox from the world. It is with them that the future health of the world rests.

One of the hardest life lessons for me to learn was that some people are truly bad. Or at least they do bad things. That realization has been harder for me to comprehend than almost anything else. After all, in *Bar 7 Theater* the bad guy *always* lost. In real life many bad guys win. If you are opposite them in the game of life, you lose. Working for a decade on AIDS allowed me a unique view of the bad side of science, medicine, and politics. The evil that emerged from self-serving scientists, them-versus-us politicians, and homophobic religious leaders was most enlightening and frightening to me. Waiting for the guy on the white horse to arrive can be deadly in the midst of a vicious epidemic like AIDS. Perhaps I should have been educated by my experience with the dean at Northwestern, but I wasn't. Hard lessons come hard. Only after years of trying to placate and sidestep obstructionist or negative people have I learned to join forces with allies and confront adversity directly. If good is going to be victorious over evil, the evil must be reckoned with directly, actively, and swiftly.

Finally, not even the briefest review of critical junctures in my life would be complete without mention of my family. My parents died in the middle of my career, and I still miss them immensely. I still need to talk to them, to hear their subtle advice, to tell them what I have been doing. But they are gone. My brother Steve remains as a vestige of the original family, and his support in tough times has been of immense importance.

And then there is my family at home, my wife Karen Starko, a well-known doctor and epidemiologist in her own right, having gained fame for discovering that aspirin caused

Reyes syndrome, and my sons Oliver and Stephen. Karen has made great personal and professional sacrifices to care for me and our children. They are the real substance of my life. With all my work and accomplishment, probably little will be remembered, and all can be replaced. But these boys will be a legacy of which I will always be proud.

In reading over this chapter, I fear that I may have misled the reader of this story by giving the impression that my life and my career have been planned out, well directed, and well organized. Nothing is further from the truth. There was no plan. My parents never put high expectations in front of me. In grammar school I wanted to be a garbage man (I liked their boots) or a mechanic (I liked their tools). I went to Berkeley because my girlfriend went there. I went to Harvard because another girlfriend went there. I went to CDC for 2 years to avoid participating in the Vietnam War. And it all worked out.

POSTSCRIPT

Dr. Don Francis continues to work at Genentech developing a vaccine for AIDS. He reports that a trial vaccine has now been given to over a thousand people, with promising results. However, the lack of social commitment to undertake a full-scale evaluation remains the major stumbling block toward final development. Dr. Francis is also working with government and nongovernment organizations to stimulate vaccine development worldwide. He lives with his wife and children in northern California.

CHAPTER VI

PHYSICIAN AS HEALER, SCIENTIST, AND TEACHER

YOLANDA HUET-VAUGHN, M.D.

I grew up a child between two cultures and had the good fortune of identifying with both. My first memories are of a small village in Mexico where my father was the people's doctor and their friend. I remember the ambience — the warmth and respect mutually exchanged between my father and our neighbors and the sense of responsibility for the well-being of this community that I felt and saw in my father. I believe that it was these early memories that motivated me to be a healer.

The seeds of my present values come from the community and family I was fortunate to inherit. For as long as I can remember, respecting and caring for one another have always been integral to family life — unconscious values taught by grandparents, aunts, uncles, and parents alike and absorbed by me and my brother and sisters. This love has been a source of strength and hope and a challenge in turn to uphold my responsibilities to the people around me.

My grandfather died recently at the age of 91, and with his passing I began to reminisce about the wonderful years we shared together. I realized that there are those who have been my role models because I consciously chose them and emulated them. And then there are those who created such an imprint in my consciousness that their influence was a given, a blending of their values into the texture of my life. My father, mother, and grandfather were all such influences.

Abuelito Antonio was a joyful man who viewed the world with possibility. He was not the best businessman, but he was always cheerful and fair in his business dealings. Through my childhood and early adulthood, he ran a bus line in Mexico City, frequently exasperating various family members because of his persistence with this borderline business endeavor. I remember his quiet calm and optimism while everyone put in their two cents' worth regarding what he should be doing. He became particularly animated when dealing with two very different topics — education and the honesty/dishonesty of government. He himself had never gone beyond the formal education of grade school, yet he had a great respect for learning. He taught himself the skills needed to run a business and to some extent even learned the difficult English language. I remember to this day one of his favorite sayings: "It is not what you have that matters, but what you know and how you use your knowledge." He enthusiastically supported me in all my educational endeavors, including taking the time to teach me to swim and patiently helping me learn to drive at age 16.

Throughout his life he had numerous encounters with police and other government officials. He became animated, like a Crusader, when confronted with what he felt was corruption in public office. His concept of government was that it should exist for the good of the people and not for the self-aggrandizement of the public official. He also felt that each person had a responsibility to keep government honest. He adamantly raved against the custom of paying "*mordidas*," stating that if we wanted honest cops, we had to expect honest cops and not contribute to corruption. And he acted on his beliefs. I remember one week he disappeared for several days — at this time he was already in his 70s — only to be found in the Mexico City jail. Apparently, he had refused to pay a bribe for the right to send his bus on its usual route. On his release he seemed none the worse for wear but thoroughly incensed at what he saw as government corruption and civilian lack of responsibility. Through it all, he retained his hopeful and joy-filled view of the world, like another Spanish compatriot who jousted with windmills several centuries past, believing that each of us could make a difference.

I would say that my father, who shared only the first 20 years of my life, also tremendously influenced me. I remember his dedication to helping others, his pleasure in giving time and skills, and the respect he had for all he cared for. My mother and her siblings, especially my Tia Licha, and my grandmother Clotilde very quietly and actively nurtured the expansion of my horizon through education.

Born in Mexico and raised after the age of 4 as an immigrant to the United States, I grew up between cultures, a part of both American and Mexican society but never 100% accepted or grounded in either. On the one hand, I was always keenly aware of the need to do well in all endeavors and of the pride of my entire family in my accomplishments. These were "our" accomplishments and a small victory over the stereotypes held by many Americans about Mexicans. On the other hand, I became enamored of the ideals of religious and political freedom and equality embodied in the U.S. Constitution and espoused by such great Americans as Martin Luther King, Jr., Cesar Chavez, Elizabeth Blackwell, Elizabeth Cady Stanton, and Harriet Tubman.

The greater portion of my grade school days were spent in the hills of Appalachia. I came as an outsider with my family into a close-knit community that I grew to love dearly. A small Catholic school provided my formal education in a building that housed the first eight primary grades within four classrooms. About a dozen students were in my class; every other year my brother's class shared my assigned teacher and room. The one difficult aspect of my life in Appalachia was that I had come from a culture in which Catholicism was a given to one where my faith made me a minority to be mistrusted and disliked. As I looked beyond the confines of my small community, I found myself in a society that emphasized the "me" outside of the context of "we" and presented success in terms of personal financial gain and achievement.

My parents provided a loving, nurturing home and a close-knit extended family. My Catholic faith reinforced a world view in which each of us was responsible for the spiritual and physical well-being of the other — a world view that defined all peoples as extended family. I read about the lives of many holy people who had placed the well-being of others ahead of their own and, as a result, had changed a small section of the world for the better. I remember reading about the woman who founded the Sisters of Charity in the United States, about St. Martin de Porres, about Dr. Tom Dooley and Dr. Albert Schweitzer. My views at that point were guided by an innate sense of compassion nurtured by family and faith.

For as long as I can remember, I knew that I would be a doctor. Strangely, it was this aspiration that initially placed me in conflict with my society. Although this was the second half of the 20th century, the idea of a girl growing up to be a doctor was still unusual and generally discouraged. It seemed unjust that I should be faced with obstacles to going to medical school simply because I was a woman. Likewise, it seemed unjust and hypocritical for the same church that nurtured my compassion and responsibility for others to place its women in what felt like second-class citizenship. Again I found myself a woman-girl between cultures, this time not between national or ethnic groupings but between the culture of patriarchy and the ideal of equality.

And so I learned to become a fighter, first as a Mexican within an Anglo culture, then as a Catholic within a Protestant society, and last as a woman within a patriarchal structure. It was in this context that I experienced the call to justice building, in particular focusing on the equitable distribution of resources in a world of a few haves and a multitude of have-nots. As I grew, and I saw the contradictions within my community grow, I did not reject my community but rather challenged it to reflect and change.

But I had no intellectual skills at this point, just the desire to serve and a gut reaction that said "to love and serve others is to live life fully." I was a bright girl, and although my parents provided me with an education, much of my learning had been by rote and not by reasoning. I have the Jesuits to thank for beginning me on the path to intellectual questioning and reasoning. In particular, I have Fathers Starkloff, Blumeyer, and Lakas and my college-to-life friend Lynn. Lynn and I were two of 100 women to integrate the up-to-then male haven of Rockhurst College. I thought I knew exactly what I wanted from the college: a premed education strong in the sciences. I got much more, but not without protest initially from me. I remember discussing with Father Blumeyer my total lack of interest in taking the required philosophy and theology courses and his firm but gentle insistence that these were needed for my growth. I subsequently took numerous courses in the philosophy of science, comparative religions, phenomenology, and political philosophy.

When I graduated from Vanderbilt University, I held an interdisciplinary major in molecular biology, philosophy, and psychology that integrated the world for me. My concept of a physician included not only the act of healing but the skills and knowledge of a scientist. I reasoned that the profession at times involved a clash of paradigms and thus required both the analytical reasoning and questioning skills of a philosopher/scientist. This is still probably the hardest task for me as a physician.

Along with the development of my intellectual skills came political awareness. I might not have developed the ability to question the political context of my life in 1969 had it not been for my professors at Rockhurst, the midnight talks with Lynn, my future husband David, and the impact of the Vietnam War. I had engaged in political action prior to college as a high school student working on the United Farm Workers Grape Boycott. I remember picketing at the A&P and leafleting the morning after Senior Prom, having convinced my date to leaflet with me between prom breakfast and the afternoon prom picnic.

But I was still acting from my heart in response to the love and commitment and call to justice made by Cesar Chavez and the many farmworker organizers. I believed still that the majority of people were just. I believed that when injustice was highlighted sufficiently for all to see, then working conditions would change and the small number of unjust people would be compelled to act differently. Studying the nature of scientific revolutions and simultaneously learning about Vietnam raised my awareness about the concept of unconsciously adopted belief structures. I had supported U.S. policy in Vietnam unthinkingly. Dr. Tom Dooley impressed me with his humanitarian work as a physician, and the impact of his political perspective affected me more than I knew. In 1969, I began to question what I saw as political commentary. At Vanderbilt University I realized that I was again between cultures, this time because of my political beliefs. I now supported an end to U.S. intervention in Southeast Asia, the farm-worker boycott, and opposition to apartheid in South Africa and racism at home. I owe Vanderbilt thanks for the opportunity to develop the strength of character and commitment to persevere with an unpopular belief system and for the opportunity to develop skills of persuasion to educate others.

At Vanderbilt I became aware of a community of justice-seeking individuals who served as role models for me: Lynn

Fitch, mother, activist, and the first woman minister I ever met; Nelson Fuson, professor at Fisk University, a Quaker, and a quietly determined and dedicated gentleman in whom I saw integrity of spiritual values and public action. Joy and Les Falk, Andy and Julia Hewitt, and Father Jack Hickey all were teachers in the most literal sense.

While anticipating an August wedding with David in 1971, I lived in the dorm at Rockhurst College working as an Upward Bound counselor with inner city youth. These young people taught me the importance of seeing life through another's eyes and expressing empathy, not sympathy. I learned from these teens that hope — or the lack of it — depends on where you come from. Future aspirations are shaped in great part by role models, both positive and negative, from within communities. And the future well-being of young people depends on many factors, including access to health care providers, socioeconomic status, education, and cultural beliefs. I also realized that my ability to influence their lives for the better depended on mutual respect and an effort to understand their reality. This was a lesson I learned many times over throughout my occupational endeavors, whether driving a cab in Kansas City, building Peterbilt trucks in Nashville, or working with seasonal and migrant farm-workers in Tennessee. Respect and understanding of the context in which an individual functioned was key to reaching out in a healing way.

The year following college I worked with a program serving seasonal and migrant workers in Tennessee. I traveled about a thousand miles per month visiting county judges, farmers, and farm-workers. I learned patience. I was forced to contain anger aroused by the living conditions I saw. Only by exercising restraint could I be effective in helping improve the educational and occupational opportunities of the farm-workers and their children. I had to diplomatically request permission from growers to go on their land to speak to workers and their families, and present county officials with program suggestions or requests for their participation and intervention.

I began to think then in terms of structures. Helping to get one child medical attention was important, but creating a structure that provided access to health care for all would ultimately improve each individual child's well-being. It was at this point that I met Joy and Les Falk. As I observed their commitment to reaching out to individuals and to molding and changing community structures, I gained a new appreciation for what I wanted to do as a doctor. Les Falk was Chairman of the Department of Family and Community Medicine at Meharry Medical College in Nashville, Tennessee, then one of two minority medical schools in the country. He introduced me to Meharry, and in 1975 I started medical school there.

Before this encounter, I had begun to wonder whether I would find anyone within the established medical profession that could appreciate my perspective. When I was a premed student at Vanderbilt, my advisor had suggested that I learn from one of his heroes and become more like Richard Nixon. I recall being pleased that I had made a 97% on an organic chemistry test, only to be chastised by this same advisor for spending my lunch hour distributing the Pentagon Papers and Amnesty International materials instead of improving my grade to 100%. I recall my interview at Kansas University. I decided that I would not gloss over who I was or what I wanted a medical school to teach me beyond the basic and clinical sciences. And thus, I went to the interview with a United Farm-Workers Boycott Grapes button pinned to my dress. When asked, I responded openly about my concerns for economic justice in relationship to the United Farm-Workers' struggle for a healthier life and how I saw this within the realm of community medicine. I was married at the time, and one of the male physicians asked me how I planned to be a wife, mother, and physician at the same time, and did I not see a conflict here? I recall explaining that there was no conflict and then at the end of the interview posing a question of my own. "Why had a similar question not been asked of the two male premed students interviewed with me, i.e., 'How did they plan on combining the roles of husband, father, and physician?'" The woman physician smiled appreciatively as the two male physician interviewers skirted around the question.

When I met Les and Joy Falk, I was living in a community that still had not outgrown its institutionalized racist roots. Vanderbilt students and faculty were only beginning to recognize the terms "sexism" and "chauvinism," much less understand them, and on the whole fully supported United States intervention in Southeast Asia. The Falks were a breath of fresh air. She was a courageous woman able to pursue her own personal agenda and at the same time empower those around her. He was a man of integrity and insight, who combined his vision of medicine with economic and social justice. Both were conscientious parents of a lovely grown family at the time of our meeting. As professor of family medicine, he helped to broaden the understanding of many future doctors. Through Les I learned about Meharry Medical School's motto: "*Servientos Mundo Deaicamus Nos Servilio Dei*" — "Worship of God Through Service to Man." And I saw the composition of the student body: 50% women, 80% black, and about 20% Hispanic, Asian-American, Native American, and white American. Meharry had a tremendous impact on my world view and my understanding of life. It was a relief to find a medical school striving for academic excellence while struggling to empower individuals and communities in their quest for physical, mental, and spiritual well-being. Thanks to Les, what I had intuitively come to understand as my role as physician was brought into focus by both faculty and classmates at Meharry and, in particular, by the Department of Family and Community Medicine.

Like Vanderbilt, Meharry also presented many challenges. Despite the common thread of service to community shared by my classmates, we were by no means a homogeneous group. The struggle to understand and respect each other was a daily one. And although Meharry allowed for a more expanded definition of the physician's role, not all my classmates shared this view. I was brought face to face with the choice of remaining silent or speaking out and facing hostile peers whose opinions in other areas I respected. For example, it was difficult for many of my male counterparts to understand why a small group of female students was interested in organizing a chapter of the American Medical Women's Association (AMWA). Despite the fact that Meharry was ahead of its time in accepting women students, the struggle of women for recognition, respect, and equal treatment with their male peers was active at my alma mater, as it was within the rest of society. It was not without some trepidation that a group of us organized a chapter of AMWA. In the face of criticism, we gathered as women to support each other and promote an understanding of the sexism within our medical school experience.

In my second year, the United States invited South Africa to participate in the Davis Cup tennis tournament, and Vanderbilt University was selected as the site for the games. My husband David and I helped to organize the Tennessee Coalition against Racism and Apartheid. We met with the Vanderbilt Chancellor to discuss the inappropriateness of Vanderbilt hosting South Africa in violation of the international sports boycott against apartheid. When Vanderbilt failed to see that hosting South Africa tacitly approved its apartheid system, we worked with justice-minded community leaders to organize visible and strong support for those in the struggle to end apartheid. Three days of demonstrations ensued. Students, laborers, professionals, blacks, whites, people from all sections of the country arrived at the Vanderbilt gymnasium in a show of solidarity.

I was on my surgery rotation at the culmination of our organizing efforts. Standing up against apartheid in South

Africa and racism here at home seemed a logical step toward improving the health and well-being of my local community as well as our world community. But I had to make a choice: participate in the one-to-one care of patients on surgery or continue with the task of trying to create a paradigm shift within a racist system. I chose to drop surgery, after transferring care of my patients, to focus on healing a social disease. Following the demonstrations, I organized and coordinated a United Nations Conference on Sports, Racism and Apartheid, cohosted by the United Nations Committee against Apartheid and Meharry Medical College. I failed to pass surgery and had to repeat the rotation later. But I am quite certain that I made the correct choice, difficult though it was. And I give credit to Meharry for providing the flexibility for me to incorporate political action within my repertoire of health-promoting tools.

While at Vanderbilt and Meharry, I became familiar with the work of a number of contemporary physicians, teachers, and artists. I met Dr. Benjamin Spock and learned of his vocal opposition to the Vietnam War and the nuclear arms buildup. He recounted how the first moratorium on above-ground testing had gained public support, in part, because of the educational efforts of physicians across the country. Children were becoming ill and dying of radiation-induced cancers. Instead of just treating case after case, doctors began to ask "Why?" They demonstrated that strontium 90 from radioactive fallout did indeed become incorporated in the deciduous teeth of children through the food chain. Pediatricians nationwide gathered and analyzed these teeth. And for these public health efforts, Dr. Spock and others were vilified in the mass media. However, he had the courage of his convictions and the knowledge of a scientist. He persevered as an educator of the community in order to change both attitudes and public policy, thus affecting health positively.

I looked for a residency program that would further my understanding of the impact of societal structures and cultural values on health, and I found the Social Medicine Family Practice program at Montefiore Hospital and Medical Center in the Bronx. There I met Victor Sidel, at the time Chair of the Department of Social Medicine. He combined the skills of social researcher, scientist, and teacher and had the courage to address public health questions in arenas not commonly identified within the realm of medicine. His discipline, productivity, and academic excellence made a venture considered by many as political into a legitimate physicians' concern. My sister Rocio, then president of American Medical Student Association (AMSA), worked with Vic on a number of projects, and in time Vic became a family friend as well as teacher, role model, and mentor.

Three other physicians have had a great impact on me. Helen Caldicott, with her energy and strong commitment to the preservation of this planet, taught me that emotional investment in an issue was not always negative. She taught me that a mother's commitment to the future of her children has a place in the practice of medicine. As physicians, we need to see all children as our children, and we must have the strength and zeal of a mother as we speak on their behalf and work to secure a healthy future for them.

I met Charlie Clements at my first AMSA convention. He was head of the International Committee, in charge of preceptorships around the world. Our first discussion, if I recall correctly, was one in which we found ourselves on opposite sides of an issue. As a representative for the Meharry chapter, I voiced concern about AMSA's preceptorship in South Africa, which in essence accepted the apartheid structure because students could not participate without regard to color. I insisted that the appropriate strategy would be to inform the preceptors that, until the system changed, AMSA could not send students to South Africa. Charlie maintained that we had to accept the structures dictated by other countries but that this did not mean we supported them. In fact, his hope was that exposure to people who opposed apartheid might result in thought-provoking discussions that would generate change in the system. What struck me about the encounter occurred when was that both of us remained respectful throughout. Another memorable encounter: Charlie had succeeded as President of AMSA in negotiating with a major bank to get Visa cards for all medical students. This was not a small feat at the time and pleased all students because it would make traveling to residency interviews less difficult. As Meharry chapter president, I suggested that we decline the bank's offer because we opposed apartheid and could not support companies that did business with South Africa. There was heated debate on the floor regarding this quandary. On the one hand, the Visa cards looked good — very good — to students who would be unable to get them on their own. On the other hand, AMSA had voted on an earlier motion presented by Meharry to publicly voice opposition to South Africa's apartheid system. Charlie had not considered this dilemma during his negotiation for the cards, but now that the conflict had been presented, he spoke up before a crowd of hundreds and suggested that we not accept the cards. He advised going on record with the bank, one of the top three doing business in South Africa, as opposing racism and apartheid. He suggested we tell the bank that as soon as they divested we would be glad to proceed with the business deal. The vote on the floor that followed was testimony that medical students can act altruistically even if it opposes their financial self-interest.

Charlie and I have since become good friends. He has steadfastly lived his beliefs, from the day he refused to fly B-52 bombing missions over Vietnam while an Air Force pilot to his commitment to the people of Central America. During the war in El Salvador, Charlie organized a health care system in the countryside and spent almost 2 years easing suffering and fighting political oppression.

I started out this chapter defining what I see as a physician's responsibilities and roles. Perhaps the person who in the last 9 years of my life has most helped me to focus on these responsibilities has been my partner and friend, Lydia Moore. She has taught a succession of medical students as well as her patients. She not only conveyed the facts of medicine but, through example, taught her students to respect the uniqueness of every person. She had a full measure of compassion for her patients, staff and colleagues. At the same time, she challenged all to be a part of the team that empowered patients to better care for themselves. At a time when patient care responsibilities were overwhelming, Lydia balanced her commitment to changing community structures with one-to-one patient encounters. She worked on the issue of violence in the community, committed her time to peace work and justice, and quietly challenged her community to look honestly at itself and change for the better. She has been a scientist and academician in her study and treatment of AIDS and other diseases, but has always remained open to the possibility that compassion and caring and humor and joy not only contribute to but are necessary for well-being and health, albeit not quantifiable. She has lived a simple life, a centered life, and a life of courage, and she has been a loyal friend when it would have been easier for her to distance herself from my notoriety.*

During medical school, I joined the Army National Guard, committing to a 7-year stint in exchange for a direct commission as a Second Lieutenant. My motivation was complicated. As a peace activist during the Vietnam War era, my love of country was frequently challenged, and the attitude "love it or leave it" translated as "agree to support policy or get labeled as anti-American." Joining the military was a way of shattering that false belief; it emphasized that due respect for the American ideals of freedom and justice went hand in hand with acting responsibly to educate others about what I

---

*Lydia Moore was killed in an automobile accident during the summer of 1994.

saw as the destructive U.S. policy in Southeast Asia. Now that the treaty was signed and U.S. troop withdrawal was accomplished, I had great hopes that I would be able to "serve my country and still serve justice." Vietnam, in my opinion, was behind us, and I presumed that the lessons of that conflict were clear to all.

Coinciding with my enlistment was the struggle to pass the Equal Rights Amendment (ERA). I strongly supported the ERA and was amazed at opposition to it during discussions on the subject. Inevitably the subject of women in the military was the trump played by those who opposed the ERA, either with dismay at the logical end result of women being drafted or with the angry retort "You women want all the rights and none of the responsibilities of equal citizenship — i.e., you wouldn't want to be drafted." I realized that in our "protected" status our opinions were discounted by policymakers and communities alike. Had women been drafted for Vietnam, I thought, we could have resisted the draft alongside our male colleagues and impacted the political arena with voices that would have been heard. We would no longer be invisible. Perhaps that war would have been over long before the casualty list reached 50,000 Americans and a million Southeast Asians. And so, in part, joining the military was a statement: "Yes, I am willing to serve equally as a responsible citizen and I make no apologies for demanding the equal rights due me as a citizen and the 'visibility' that comes with equality."

I was also a medical student in need of clinical experience and on my own financially. The military promised to provide me with experience doing physical exams under the preceptorship of an established physician. At the same time, the military would provide me with a part-time job one weekend a month, and though not providing a great salary, they provided flexibility: if I couldn't make a drill because of exams or medical call I would be excused.

At that time in my life, I was not a pacifist. I believed in fighting for my values, although my concept of fighting was one of political and spiritual struggle and not military combat. Like so many of my generation I honored the warrior, and yet I could not join the military as a combatant. What was honorable about the warrior was his or her willingness to risk self for a greater good or ideal. This self-sacrifice was similar to that of the early Christians and a view I had honored as a child. It is strange, in retrospect, how the common thread of commitment took me from nonviolent martyr and pacifist to the militarism of 20th century America in the blink of an eye, with the sanctions and encouragement of most of our Christian establishment.

I should mention here that there were several "pacifist" Christians whom I met during my undergraduate years at Vanderbilt who greatly influenced me, though it was not so apparent at the time. These include Nelson Fuson and his wife Marion Fuson, members of the Society of Friends; Anderson Hewitt, and Julia Cuervo Hewitt who headquartered the draft counseling office in their home; and Jack Hickey, Catholic chaplain and founder of Dismas House. I also had become aware of the educational work of an organization called the American Friends Service Committee (AFSC). As I matured, the integrity of values and action of these friends became clear to me. Ultimately, their example and those of a handful of others encouraged me to risk the action I took in 1992.

But back to my "military" career. Once in the military, I proceeded with the assumption that the United States was benevolent, although occasionally misguided. I had been interviewed by Army Intelligence from Ft. Campbell during one of my first drills and questioned about my political activities and beliefs from 1969 to the mid-1970s. I was very candid.

I presumed that this was part of the initiation process but later found out that Army Intelligence officers met with none of the other recruits. For almost 2 hours I answered questions posed by the two officers. My views on the Vietnam War and my involvement as coordinator/chairperson for the

Nashville Peace Coalition were discussed. My concerns regarding international law and the Geneva Accords were made known, and I applauded those Vietnam vets who refused orders that violated human rights. In my innocence, I presumed that the military of a democracy looked for honorable people of conscience who would have the courage to stand up for their beliefs, and not automatons who would follow each and every order. The interview ended after queries about my membership in certain organizations on a long list. By the third or fourth organization, I recognized the list as the House Un-American Activities list of subversive organizations. I advised the Army Intelligence officers that this manner of testing was illegal but that I had no problem continuing if they wished. The interview came to an abrupt end with their flushed cheeks and "hems" and "haws." When I asked them why I had been interviewed, they responded that they needed to make sure I wasn't interested in the violent overthrow of the government. Unbeknownst to me, until February 1992, these same intelligence officers questioned faculty and classmates at my medical school about me. I remained in the Army Guard/Reserves for 5 of the 7 years to which I had committed. In my second year of residency, my reserve unit sent me to a conference on nuclear, biological, and chemical warfare and the medical response.

Early in the course of discussing the effects of nuclear weapons, the presenter made a grossly erroneous statement. I was well versed in the topic, as I had just organized a local chapter of Physicians for Social Responsibility in Kansas City and had done hours of public education on the subject of the medical response to nuclear war. I raised my hand and proceeded to provide the accurate information. A half-dozen quiet, polite corrections later, the presenter finally looked at me and said, "Look lady, I'm not advocating a nuclear war, I'm just trying to do my job." To which I replied, "But your job is giving us misinformation." A half-dozen doctors and nurses came up afterwards to thank me for my comments. I was dismayed that in the guise of medical education deliberate misinformation was being provided. And I realized that, especially in this setting, my colleagues deserved an honest and nonmanipulative presentation of data. Dr. Helen Caldicott had shown me how knowledge and commitment could help create a more life-engendering paradigm for our world. Her sense of urgency, her courage and optimism, and her perseverance motivated me to bring the ideas of nuclear disarmament to my Army colleagues and to my community.

When I resigned my commission in the Army in 1982, I requested a deferral of the last two years of my commitment in order to complete my United States Public Health Service scholarship obligation. I presumed that the deferment had been granted when I received an honorable discharge. In the ensuing years, I became increasingly critical of United States foreign policy, and although now out of the USPHS, I did not return to the Army Reserves for fear of finding myself with conflicting responsibilities. When the Berlin Wall came down, I felt hopeful that the elimination of nuclear weapons would be possible. In addition, the rationale of fighting the Soviets throughout the world was no longer applicable. Thus, I felt the use of our military would be for legitimate defense. Given these circumstances and a sense of obligation to complete the last 2 years of my 7-year commitment, I rejoined the Army Reserves in the summer of 1990. In August 1990, Saddam Hussein invaded Kuwait, the U.S. military arrived in Saudi Arabia, and I found myself in opposition to a military resolution of the conflict.

The three drills that I participated in before being called to active duty were occasions for discussion. I challenged the veracity of the information being transmitted to us by the President. I read extensively and could not find any evidence for the "domino theory" — first Kuwait, then Saudi Arabia, then the rest of the Middle East falling to Iraq. I felt using American forces to gain control of Middle Eastern oil was a gross abuse of military personnel and a violation of the Constitution. And I sensed no sincerity in George Bush's attempts to resolve the crisis. Rather, I became convinced that the President's agenda was for war. The bellicose manner with which he approached any discussions with the "other" was more and more clear as the days melted into weeks. He refused even to use the term "negotiate" in reference to Saddam Hussein.

In reacting to this purely militaristic approach, I was forging a new value within myself as conscientious objector. In the fall of 1990, I was what could be termed a "selective conscientious objector," opposed to participation in a military project for ethical reasons that did not include opposition to the use of force in and of itself. However, my experience tempered my values. I became aware of a vaccination program that I, as a physician, would be asked to participate in. The vaccines approved for the military were *Botulinum* toxoid and anthrax vaccines. The FDA had "waived" a physician's responsibility to provide informed consent to those he or she would order to be inoculated. I felt this policy not only violated international law and the Nuremberg Code but profoundly breached my trust with the troops I was responsible for. I was aware that 60,000 body bags had been sent to the Gulf, that our medical teams' rescue efforts would have shortcomings, and that many of our troops would be "triaged in the sand" in case of an all-out ground war. How could I, in good faith, pretend to all those under my care that everything was under control when in fact I knew it was not? How could I, in good faith, lend my efforts to a military solution that would leave, by conservative estimates 50,000 to 100,000 civilian casualties in a country where over 50% of the population was under the age of 15 years? These were questions that kept going through my mind as I received orders to report to active duty.

I reported to duty and every step of the way voiced my objections. I pointed out that we had deployed over 400 nuclear weapons to the Gulf. These weapons were weapons of mass destruction targeting not only a military force but the civilian population and the environment. I stated that I could not support this policy and would have to speak out against the deployment of these weapons. I initially hoped that I could "go along" with the program, as I did not believe that the President would choose war without truly exhausting other options. However, President Bush finally convinced me that he had no interest in anything other than a military solution. When I saw that he was willing to gamble the lives of American troops and Iraqi civilians and risk catastrophic environmental consequences like the oil well fires (which had been predicted in November 1990 at a United Nations conference on the environment), I knew that I had a responsibility to attempt to impact policy through public education. The war at this point was still preventable. I sought advice from my husband David and from Charlie Clements, Bill Monning, and Vic Sidel. As I mentioned earlier, Charlie had refused to undertake bombing missions during the Vietnam War — for this he was placed in psychiatric facilities for over a year and ultimately discharged from the service. Bill was Executive Director of the International Physicians for the Prevention of Nuclear War (IPPNW) and very knowledgeable about international law and the catastrophic consequences of a Gulf War. But most important, he was a caring and committed person trying to make a difference for the better. I discussed the dilemma I faced. Their support made my options clearer and helped me to delineate my responsibilities.

Ultimately, I made the decision to leave my military post and speak publicly about the catastrophic consequences of a military resolution. I read a poem by Gary Sugarman, a poem I carried around in my wallet for a number of years. In that poem the poet talks about the simple peoples of this earth who have no voice in this, the animals and trees who have no voice, and the children who have no voice. And he hoped that those of us who could speak, those of us who could make a difference in support of all those with no voice, that those of us who could speak prove worthy of this trust. I looked at a picture of my children's faces and they blurred into faces of Iraqi, Israeli, and Saudi children, and I felt the pain and terror of those Middle Eastern mothers who were voiceless except in their mourning. I saw myself as one of them. And I hoped that those who could make a difference in preserving my children's lives and futures would act to prevent the impending disaster. The choice was very simply made at that point. My children . . . their children . . . these were all our children.

POSTSCRIPT

As a result of Dr. Huet-Vaughn's refusal to support the Gulf War, she was charged by the United States Military with desertion with the intent to avoid important and hazardous service. She was sentenced to 3 years at Leavenworth, a maximum-security military prison. One month into her internment, Amnesty International declared Dr. Huet-Vaughn a "Prisoner of Conscience" and initiated a wide-scale campaign on her behalf. She was released in April, 1992 after 8 months of imprisonment. A long series of appeals and reconsiderations of her case in military court is still under-way. Based on Dr. Huet-Vaughn's "unprofessional conduct," the Kansas Board of Healing Arts considered revoking her medical license but finally dropped the case after 2 years.

Dr. Huet-Vaughn currently works as a family practitioner at Family Health Services in Kansas City, Kansas. This clinic serves many of the city's low-income and minority groups, including its sizable Hmong community. She is also on the faculty at one of Kansas City's Family Practice residency programs and helps staff that hospital's infectious disease clinic.

CHAPTER VII

THE PERSPECTIVE OF DETACHMENT; THE DETACHMENT OF PERSPECTIVE

NOEL SOLOMONS, M.D.

I recommend the condition of detachment, yes detachment even to the point of alienation, as a perspective to see clearly the world around one. And possibly, I might add, to see the formative aspects of one's own life. I write this narrative largely from Guatemala, where I have been an expatriate for the past 18 years. It is a given that I travel a great deal; theories on the origins of this *Wanderlust* are discussed later on. Suffice it to say that I remember clearly my first realization of the value of detachment in seeing things clearly; it came in the spring of 1970. I was then in my final year of Harvard Medical School and had opted to take a research elective at the Universidad del Valle in Cali, Colombia.

It was during that time that President Nixon, in his wisdom, had decided to enlarge the conflict in Indochina with incursions into Laos and the bombing of the Ho Chi Minh Trail; it was during that time that students at Kent State University, in their enthusiasm, decided to protest this escalation to the war in Vietnam; it was during that time that the National Guardsmen of the state militia of Ohio, in their patriotism, decided to mow their fellow citizens down with gunfire. Stunned — but not surprised — I read news from the international wire services in Colombia's dailies. The naked reality of what Kent State meant was unelaborated and unembellished. I remember thinking how differently the news might impact those watching Huntley–Brinkley or Walter Cronkite, where the Kent State story was sandwiched between briefs from the Mekong Delta and the Major League baseball scores. This was America — not only at war with the "spread of Communism," not only at war with the Vietnamese peasant, but at war with itself. And living in the Valle del Cauca of Colombia gave me the detatchment to truly understand.

This was not the first revelation that had come to me in a Latin American country, nor would it be the last. Three years before the Kent State events, I had been on a pediatric malnutrition metabolic ward and research unit at the Anglo-American Hospital in Lima, Peru. I was not only away from the United States for the first time in my 22 years of life but on practically my first sojourn outside of New England. What I discovered would wed me firmly to the goal of an expatriate life-style. For the first time, I realized that I could be seen simply as a fellow human being by other human beings — Peruvian co-workers in this instance. They looked at, and found, the *person* behind the black skin that was the heritage of my birth in Boston on New Year's Eve, 1944. It was not that Peruvians did not know racism; the schism that separates descendants of the indigenous Inca from those of the Spaniard is long and deep. To my good fortune, however, they did not know North American racism. I could be seen as a person! It was an intellectual revelation as well as a feeling and an experience too precious ever to relinquish.

Recently, as I was viewing a broadcast with footage from the March on Washington for Jobs and Freedom of 1963, my mind was drawn to another important insight gained August 28, 1963, the day of the march, during the bus ride back up Interstate 95. That night I chatted with a psychiatry resident at the Massachusetts Mental Health Center, a self-avowed "white liberal," who described going out of his way to treat black patients with more compassion and skill than the white patients. When dissatisfied with treatment, the resident's white patients would blame it directly on him; a black patient would resolve the same quandary by blaming it on his or her race.

My traveling companion described the concept of a shell — a "defense mechanism" — that defends blacks from the agony of determining whether we were being viewed through the prism of another's racial reflex. So for security's sake, we assume skin color always factors into others' reactions to us. Period! In this brief narrative, raised to defuse the tension between us, Dr. Zonana explained me. There was peace and resignation in recalling that moment when a concept, "black paranoia," gave a Harvard undergraduate words for his chronic, life-long angst. It would be 4 years later, among the house staff and nurses of a Peruvian pediatrics department, that I would find a scenario by which the person could be seen, where the defenses had no resonance. Of course, the scenario involved being somewhere other than the United States.

Going back to the liberating moment of realization in Peru in 1967, one can understand the decision for expatriate residence in a foreign land. The push–pull paradigm of repulsion from New England's racist climate and the pull of a place where "personhood" could be experienced cemented a tour of duty into a prolonged residence. Baldwin wrote his

Notes of a Native Son from France; I write mine from Central America.

Initially, I was estranged from the terms of the invitation to contribute to this volume, a reaction probably common to many. "Me, a 'physician–activist'?!?!" I *was* an activist, but that was long ago. But I am doubly fortunate. My tool of detachment allows me to see our editor's term through my own prism, and the strains of *We Shall Overcome* have reconnected me to my activism. In Spanish we call this a *conyuntura,* a sort of a coincidence, but with celestial overtones.

THE BEGINNING BEFORE THE BEGINNING

Well, what do you know about me by now? By the context of this book, you know I am a physician. From the foregoing section, you may have divined that I am black, a native Bostonian, a veteran of the Civil Rights Movement, a nutritionist, an academic, a world traveler, and a Spanish-speaking expatriate living in Guatemala. As to my sex, "Noel" is a somewhat gender-neutral first name; but if you know anything about Harvard Medical School's admission policies in the 1970s, or that Harvard College and Radcliffe were very separate entities in the late 1960s, those clues would suffice to establish that I am also male.

To take the advice of the Caterpillar to Alice, I shall begin at the beginning. I was born into a family of black middle-class professionals. My mother (Olivia) was a teacher who graduated from Cambridge Latin School, Salem Normal School, and Boston University, and my father (Gustave) was an electrical engineer who graduated from Quincy High School and M.I.T. In 1928, he was the only black in his graduating class. Their social network of black (Scottish) freemasons, black Greek-letter sorority (Alpha Kappa Alpha) and fraternity (Omega Psi Phi) was of a similar cultural bent.

Chosen for my godparents were a black lawyer (latter to become a juvenile court judge) and his librarian wife.

They say that with a 6-year gap between births, the second born takes on the characteristics (neurotic, driven, achieving, etc.) of a first born. So with Gus Jr., who preceded me into the world by 7 years, and me, Gus Sr. and Olivia had the equivalent of two first-born sons. My paternal grandmother passed away when I was 3; she, as well as my paternal grandfather, was born and raised on islands of the Dutch Antilles in the Caribbean. My maternal grandmother, who lived next door until her death in 1974, participated actively in my rearing. She and her late husband were migrants to Cambridge from North Carolina. Inman Street was a racially integrated street, but into number 85 had moved the Solomons family next to the Steads at 89 (there is no 87), two black families side by side in the middle of the block. Olivia and Gustave met over the back fence; that is how my mother later came to live at 85 and how my brother and I evolved as motes in our parent's eyes.

After graduating from college, my mother left "liberal" Boston and went off to teach in Greensboro, North Carolina. There she traveled the South with the school chorus and learned the reality of Jim Crow. What Woodward called "slave stigma," I would have to say applied to my late mother. Hattie McDaniel's role in *Gone with the Wind* truly troubled my mother, and she never wanted me to see that classic. My brother, today a world-famous modern dancer, was then a high school student exploring all facets of both the graphic and performing arts. At that time he was awarded the Slave Jim role in the Boston Children's Theater production of Huckleberry Finn, but Olivia insisted that "No son of mine will portray a slave." Gus Jr. declined the role.

Greensboro's Woolworth lunch counter sit-in in 1960 was another telling moment in terms of my mother's character. My first response was to ignore the call for a lunch-counter boycott. I had had a hot dog at the Woolworth's in Central

Square, Cambridge, on a weekly basis for a dozen years. My mother, having stared Jim Crow in the face, showed solidarity. "If you eat a hot dog in Woolworth's, may it stick in your craw," she said. I had a distinguished career in grammar school and high school in Cambridge, a city with relatively integrated housing patterns and multiracial schools. I was a member, over the years, of untold multiethnic groups at the YMCA, in the Boy Scouts, on sports teams, and in school activities. But I knew there were separate societies. The Bishop Rush Memorial African Methodist Episcopal Zion Church, of which my mother was an active member, represented, for me, the embodiment — and curiously, the refuge — of a black society, upstairs, in the sanctuary of the church.

The Horn twins, sons of a liberal, white Lutheran minister who had been drummed out of a Virginia church for his racial teachings, were responsible for one of my first acts of activism. Charles and Bill Horn were alternately my home room classmates and best friends during elementary and high school. Somehow, they found out about a demonstration in Lexington, Massachusetts, against a realtor who would not show houses to black families. Along with other classmates, we picketed in protest on a triangular walk beneath a flagpole with the inscription "Cradle of Liberty."

THE STUDENT ACTIVIST

At 6 feet 4 inches I was destined to be a big man on campus, but BMOC for the entering freshman class of Harvard in the autumn of 1962. About half of the students at Harvard came from prep schools, like Exeter and Andover, and this was true also of the *black* freshmen: half of them were also true preppies. This I found very interesting. I was no less immune to the hidden agenda of college life — groping for an adult identity — than anyone else.

Freshman year at Harvard led to three currents of activism. The first was the civil rights movement. The first Mississippi Freedom Summer had just concluded, and the Student Nonviolent Coordinating Committee (SNCC) had become a common word. We Bostonians were examining the issues to address at home. Discrimination issues in Greater Boston allowed for direct action by blacks and whites together, whether against housing discrimination in the suburbs, job discrimination downtown, or *de facto* segregated schools in the ghetto. The Boston Action Group (BAG), led by Noel Day, a social worker with the St. Mark's Church in Roxbury, was an eminent local direct-action group. While the NAACP was being shocked out of contemplative inaction, BAG was hitting the streets. And, along with five colleagues from Radcliffe and Harvard, I began attending the BAG meetings and actions on North Dorchester's Blue Hill Avenue. Back on the Cambridge side of the river, the Harvard–Radcliffe civil rights activists formed a biracial association on campus that became known as CRCC (to rhyme with SNCC), the Civil Rights Coordinating Committee. I knew it intimately, as I became its first chairman.

The number of black faces on the greater Harvard campus was increasing, and with the appointment of Dr. Harold Amos in the medical school, Harvard even had a tenured black professor! Africa's decolonization had significant cultural effects on America's black population, manifesting itself in terms of garb — the dashiki, the tricolored (black, red, green) banners and skull caps — and the Afro hairdo. The real aficionado was reading the poetry of Ghana's Kwami Nkruma on "negritude" while maintaining James Baldwin's *Go Tell It on the Mountain* on the night table. The message of the Honorable Elijah Mohammed and the Muslims was making its way to my consciousness through *Ebony* and *Jet,* reaching the at-large population later through the voice of Malcolm X, a Boston native. Many of us of black pigmentation — both African students and Afro-American students —

practiced exclusivity by contemplating and discussing matters with ourselves, by ourselves. This led to the organizing of the AAAAS, the Association of African and Afro-American Students, at Harvard and Radcliffe. Through shame, guilt, curiosity, or attraction, the nascent AAAAS actually succeeded in getting almost 100% of the black students and faculty into the same salon on several Sundays during my first two collegiate years.

"Enlightened" Harvard had rules against discrimination in membership of its officially sanctioned clubs and organizations, so the focus and rules of the AAAAS were viewed as discriminatory. Interestingly, I found myself having to attack race-based discrimination within CRCC while defending racial separation in justifying the membership exclusivity of the AAAAS. The college experience was forming an agile mind.

My third thread of activism became manifest in relation to early opposition to U.S. militarism in Indochina. By the spring of 1963, there was nothing like a good demonstration. I joined about 20 other marchers at the entrance to the Harvard Square subway entrance on May 2 in the first national antiwar demonstration. It was not so much my campus colleagues but a high school classmate, Abbie Schirmer, who raised my consciousness on this issue. The new comrades I made on May 2 led me to affiliation with Harvard Radcliffe's Socialist Club, which was headed by an intense student named Henry Kahn, and later to the Cambridge version of the Students for a Democratic Society. Interestingly, there was broad cross-registration in CRCC and the SDS. By the time I ascended Bus 17 for the trip to Washington in August of 1963, I was partaking in the activism of the mainstream civil rights movement, the ideology of the New Left, and the critical reflection of the culture of negritude.

My grade-point average was well maintained. I pursued a concentration major in biochemical sciences and followed up on my high school avocations. I tried out for glee club and did not make it; I tried out for the Freshman intercollegiate basketball team and did not make it; I tried out for the Harvard Band and was welcomed. There was not a week that did not see me leading or attending one or another political meeting, nor a month that did not find me canvassing or picketing. I had the opportunity to dine with Dr. Martin Luther King when the Young Democrats invited him to Harvard for a speech, and to speak to James Baldwin when the AAAAS sponsored him in Sanders Theater.

The most memorable moment of the student activist days (after the March on Washington, of course) came in 1964 in the nationwide support of the marchers in Selma, Alabama. To stop the brutality of Sheriff "Bull" Conner, those who could not be at the head of the bridge in Selma took to the Federal Buildings around the country. Protesters took to sitting inside these buildings and singing "We shall not be moved," until President Johnson and the Justice Department sent in federal marshals. Over the 3 days, representatives from all of the eastern colleges occupied the upper floor of the granite building overlooking Congress Square until the sought-after federal marshals deposited us unceremoniously on the cold sidewalks outside. We experienced a deep solidarity of purpose and communion. Tears came to my eyes as I saw the host of friends on the picket lines beneath, unable to gain access to the building once it has been cordoned off.

Activism shaped my road to physicianhood in a textured and multifaceted way. The State Department had realized around 1965, no doubt after having watched me and 250,000 other people marching close to Foggy Bottom in the March on Washington, that of 1600 Foreign Service Officers, only 36 were black. They began a crash program in affirmative action, and a recruiter came to the Harvard campus. Dean Archie Epps contacted some of the juniors in the AAAAS, and after my 20 years of confinement in New England, I was itching for some geographic diversity. I applied and was accepted. As a science major, the State Department placed me on the seventh floor (Secretary's level) of the New State Building in the Office of Science and Technology. Even summer interns get background checks for security clearances, but my top-floor assignment required a Top Secret clearance. As word of my civil rights, SDS, and antiwar inclinations filled the reviewer's file, my clearance possibilities plummeted. (This I learned from the manager of the program.) So my assignment changed to a small office of health affairs in the Agency for International Development, where a Confidential clearance was all that was necessary.

On the seventh floor, I would have worked on the diplomatic issues related to a satellite falling from the sky and injuring someone in another country. In the basement of the Annex building, I was assigned to do a literature review concerning the interaction of malnutrition and mental development. USAID was besieged by suitors for funds to support studies addressing the relationship between permanent cognitive incapacitation and episodes of severe protein–energy malnutrition. There was a literature, much of it not in English, and my job was to find it, cite it, and review it. The final paper, *Food for Thought,* was the product of many trips to the George Washington and National Medical Library.

As interns, we attended assembly briefings by Ambassador Averill Harriman. I remember how he and others were assailed with pointed questions from the college students in the audience; clearly, I was not the only one with anti-Vietnam War sentiments. One day we were called to the auditorium, where we listened solemnly to President Johnson's announcement committing 500,000 men to Vietnam. This would be a significant summer. On the political front, antiwar feelings superseded the civil rights agenda for me. How could I live in (much less work for the diplomacy arm of) a country that would do what the United States was doing in Vietnam? Could I find *any* profession or pursuit that was not intrinsically corrupt? In my summer exposures, I found answers. The people working on the nutrition–mental development question worked abroad. They gave food to children. What could be more essentially apolitical and intrinsically good than addressing malnutrition? I decided first to become a physician, this so I could become a public health physician, this so I could become a worker in international nutrition, and this so I could live away from the United States. I wanted to be dissociated from the U.S. neocolonialist policies and to be detached from its subsoils. I also had an urge to see face to face these exotically named malnutrition syndromes "kwashiorkor" and "marasmus."

THE PHYSICIAN–ACTIVIST

Since Harvard Medical School treated us as "young physicians" from the time we first donned white coats, I shall date the period of my physician activism from entrance to medical school. Fervor for political activism had preceded me to the Longwood Avenue campus, as Henry Kahn was in his third year at HMS when I entered in 1966. The Student Health Organization was growing across the nation's medical schools. New York, Detroit, Chicago, and Boston had potent branches with seasoned Movement veterans in leadership positions. To some extent, the SHO was an offspring of the Medical Committee for Human Rights. However, by 1966, SHO had gone beyond civil rights movement concerns to concentrate on the war in Vietnam and reform of the medical profession. The organization was analyzing the economics of health care and the plight of the poor. With three medical schools, two dental schools, and a plethora of nursing schools and allied health sciences programs in the Greater Boston area, I dedicated effort to recruiting students and proselytizing on other campuses to get the "uninitiated" into the fold.

I shall never forget the evening in 1968 I flew into and out of Newark Airport to participate in the taping of the *David Suskind Show* on the topic "Radicals in Medical

School." I was the token Harvardian (and also the token
black) in a group that included the SHO's founding leaders
Peter Schall, Fitzhugh Mullen, and Bill Bronson. The students' analysis was truly radical and scathing: of medicine;
of politics; of society. I had a pharmacology final exam the
next morning, for which I was marginally prepared, but I
was too exhausted to return to studying. I awoke the next
morning to the news that Robert Kennedy had been shot in
California. I thought for sure the pharmacology exam would
be canceled. It was not. I did not do well in basic pharmacology.

As it turned out, I was much more active and involved
with the Medical Committee for Human Rights (MCHR)
throughout my medical school years than with the SHO. The
MCHR originally was the voluntary medical support unit for
the summer civil rights workers in the South. It was a multiracial organization, and Dr. Quentin Young of Chicago and
Dr. Walter Lear of Philadelphia were prominent in the national leadership. One superb physician whom I got to know
at the MCHR meetings was Dr. Irv Rosenberg, then an affiliate in gastroenterology at the Boston City Hospital. We
would gather for coffee breaks to talk of our Third-World experiences and even of the role of folic acid in intestinal
health. This defining paradigm of the Third World and the
gut was to have a profound influence on my research career,
as was the personal contact. I would later join Dr. Rosenberg
in Chicago to pursue my clinical research training.

Martin Luther King's murder, perhaps, wiped away any
remaining optimism I had about U.S. capacity to resolve the
"racial thing." Of course, I shared the bitterness and seething
anger that became manifest across the nation. The MCHR's
national meeting scheduled for the following day was not
called off, so I proceeded to travel to Philadelphia. Anger, dis-
traction, and deflation were my feelings at the conclave.
America had lost its conscience the day before and, for one

embittered second-year medical student, any vestige of hope
for social salvation.

In 1969, I helped organize a contingent of my classmates
to don white coats and helmets with red crosses and join in
the massive "Bring the Troops Home" march on the Pentagon.
This demonstration was second to the 1963 march only in
terms of numbers; it exceeded the latter in hostility and in
response from security, which can be summed up as tear gas,
tear gas, and more tear gas. The black bag came in handy
that afternoon; I treated a bystander provoked into a grand
mal seizure by the mace that wafted into the crowds of shop-
pers. If the Tet offensive marked the turning point of the war
in Vietnam, the March on the Pentagon marked the turning
point of the antiwar movement. Through irritated eyes and
rasping throats, we all knew that withdrawal and peace
would be only a matter of time.

I considered two training programs for internship and
residency in internal medicine after graduation. One was in
Boston at the Beth Israel Hospital; the other was at the Hospital of the University of Pennsylvania in Philadelphia. There
was cultural comfort in the Beth Israel Hospital option because many of my colleagues in the MCHR and the movement
were based at this location. But I also felt a need to get out
of Boston after 25 years, and the latter consideration won
out. I later discovered that the intern selection committee had
fiercely debated what my conduct would be if there were a
sit-in at the Cambridge campus. Would I stay at my bedside
duties or abandon my patients for the demonstration? Finally,
they agreed that I would choose the former course, and gave
me a matching rank.

In Philadelphia, my activism promptly resurfaced. This
program was based not only in the university hospital but
also in the general hospital and the Veterans' Hospital. My
terms of selection included payment by the Veterans' Administration tie-in. But this meant swearing allegiance, and I
would have none of a "loyalty oath," neither swearing nor

affirming. I was switched to university payroll and never entered the VA facility until I was a senior resident.

There is nothing like an every-third-night on-call schedule and lack of sleep to dampen one's activist fervor. I was able to wear a dashiki and white pants with my stethoscope and black bag, and the department head looked the other way. However, my attendance at demonstrations and MCHR meetings tapered off. Of course, the war persisted, as did conscription of physicians. I was called for my predraft physical examination in my internship year, but I was never called for service, so the personal issue of the act of draft refusal never came up.

My one true vacation came at the end of my internship. I made a pilgrimage to the three sites of my medical school research — Bogota, Cali, and Lima — theorizing that malnutrition and intestinal nutrient absorption formed the coming paradigm. My planning for postresidency training began to take shape; I would focus on clinical nutrition and gastroenterology. Irv Rosenberg had moved from Boston to Chicago, and together we designed a fellowship at the University of Chicago to begin in July 1973. I found the Hyde Park community to be a racial oasis; there were more interracial couples on my block than single-race dyads. However, I was quite uncomfortable with the University Hospital's juxtaposition of its South-Side neighborhood (black) inpatients and its North-Side (white) clientele.

Gastrointestinal complaints are heavily overlain with emotional distress, and vice versa. In the more relaxed setting of the clinical fellowship, I was able to get back to the principles of compassion and support for the patient, a process that was extremely satisfying. Working with patients around the issues of sexuality and self-image was a cherished and positive aspect of my Chicago phase. I finally tested our "radical" theories of physician–patient interaction that eschewed laying power trips. They worked!

THE PROFESSIONAL ACTIVIST

In the 1960s and 1970s, the mantra was "never trust anyone over 30." I understand this phrase better now: it is not maturity or conservatism that intervenes in the fourth decade but the loss of youthful energy. Coincidentally, I experienced my 40th birthday 21 days before I took up residence in Guatemala in 1985. Although I did not renounce my medical license, that date marks my transformation from "physician" to "research professional." Guatemala is a country of physical beauty, cultural richness, social turmoil, and recurrent violence. In the past 19 years, I have been touched by all of these features.

Analogous to the situation in Lima, where I encountered Peruvians unschooled in North American racism, I found myself in Guatemala without grounding in their particular brand of ethnic hostility. I accepted Mayan and Ladino alike as persons. This attitude — unusual in Guatemala — is something that all parties have observed in *gringos* over the years; they are not astounded at this eccentricity. My egalitarian point of view gained tangible form when I brought into my laboratory group the brilliant young woman, Celia Chet, a *Kakchiquel*-speaking native of San Juan Sacatepequez. Later, I accepted the responsibility to be the *padrino* (godfather) of her son, Jose Felipe Ralac Chet, the product of her marriage to Felipe Ralac, a *Quiché*-speaking bilingual educator from Momostenango. This decision had life-long implications; in 1982, political repression took Celia and Felipe away in a kidnapping and murder. I accepted the consequence of god-paternity and since that time have raised Josecito in my household as a son.

It may seem contradictory for an activist to find solace and refuge in a country renowned for violations of human rights. The social turmoil of Guatemala is fueled by a racial encounter: the confrontation of the original, indigenous post-Mayan population and the Spanish European *conquistadores*. I should make clear that the one form of activism I have avoided has been political or human rights activism of and about Guatemala. This type of activity is not viable for an expatriate and is antithetical to conducting science in an institutional context.

Inaction, however, is not necessarily equivalent to looking the other way. The progression from analysis to advocacy requires a truly profound understanding of the complexities of the consequences. It is illegal for noncitizens of Guatemala to engage in political activities, with a penalty of deportation. So, my lack of direct activism concerning human rights issues in Guatemala has a pragmatic dimension. My motivation to action and activism in the United States had been self-interest, or even self-defense. It is one thing to see the pain of racial discrimination fall on another, and yet another to feel it fall on oneself. In my life, the latter has been more motivating.

The personal relationships that I have maintained over almost 20 years in Guatemala have been drawn from four communities: from the *Ladino,* indigenous, and expatriate communities of Guatemala and from friends and colleagues in the United States and other countries. The people in this network come from a wonderful assortment of backgrounds, as the traditional bases of family, neighborhood, and social class have not been of primary importance for me. The workplace, both at the Institute of Nutrition of Central America and Panama (INCAP) and at the Center for Studies of Sensory Impairment, Aging and Metabolism (CeSSIAM), has been a source of friendships. In the *Ladino* group, physicians and scientists have made up the major constituency of close friends. Among the indigenous Guatemalans, it has been both professionals and the family of my adopted son. In the expatriate community, there are casual acquaintances in the various English-speaking establishments, with some dear friends in the private voluntary organizations. I truly have been able to maintain, and extend, close relationships — including romantic ones — in countries external to Guatemala.

My base in Guatemala from 1975 to 1985 was INCAP. It was founded by Dr. Nevin Scrimshaw in 1949 as a research outpost of the Pan American Health Organization, a United Nations agency, and was administered with policy governance from the Ministers of Health of the six republics of the isthmus. I retained a faculty appointment at Chicago, but I was a tutorial fellow with Dr. Fernando Viteri in INCAP's Biomedical Division. For the duration of my decade plus at the Institute, I was in an *ad honorem* "affiliated" position, which meant privilege but no power. The energy I previously devoted to political activism was rechanneled into perfecting my language fluency, exploring Guatemala's culture and geography, romance, and the publish-or-perish imperative of a biomedical investigator. That meant long hours on the metabolic ward, in the lab, and in the library.

Nevin Scrimshaw had moved on in 1962 to become Professor Scrimshaw and head of the Department of Nutrition and Food Science at the Massachusetts Institute of Technology. I had written my college honors thesis with him through a cross-Cambridge cross-registration arrangement. He developed a small, academic, multidiciplinary "think tank" called the International Food and Nutrition Policy Planning Program that was long on policy and planning and short on scientific nutrition. Thus, I accepted a time-sharing position as Assistant Professor in 1977 to allow for half the year teaching in Cambridge and half the year researching in Guatemala.

I would characterize myself as a clinical nutritionist and a human nutritionist, with a focus on how nutrients are absorbed into the body and on what factors impair, enhance or generally regulate the uptake of essential compounds from the diet. This has led me to an exploration of the complexity of diet and of the diseases in tropical countries (diarrhea, parasite infections) that influence intestinal health. My research along these lines has covered virtually all types of nutrients: proteins, carbohydrates, vitamin A, folic acid, iron, zinc, and selenium.

Inevitably, I became concerned with describing the nutritional situation of overall populations in developing countries. This led to an additional line of research on assessing nutritional status, in part to improve our diagnostic methods and in part to survey specific populations in Guatemala. We have worked, at CeSSIAM, with biochemical tests of nutrient reserves. In line with the cultural circumstances in developing countries, we have sought ways to avoid blood samples and to assay other body fluids such as tears or urine. The functional assessment of nutritional status, using the intactness of metabolic and physiological responses in the body, has also been a focus of my attention.

The conventional focus of nutrition research in the Third World is on rural populations and in maternal and child health. These geographic and demographic foci have saturated the agendas of most research centers in developing countries. I have taken several alternative tacks, exploring the urban population's nutrition and diet problems and looking into dimensions of aging and gerontology.

My work has taken me to all of the continents of the world. Most often, I have attended conferences and congresses to share experiences or to present data derived from studies in Guatemala. I have also had the opportunity to teach and/or collaborate on research in other localities. In the early 1980s, I was invited to Sao Paulo, Brazil, to give minicourses on basic nutrition. In the mid-1980s, the German Agency for International Cooperation (G.T.Z.) was helping to develop a Masters of Science in Nutrition program at the Federal University of Rio de Janeiro and hired me to develop and teach the module on Basic Nutrition and Nutrient Requirements. Currently, in the 1990s, I am teaching in a G.T.Z.-funded project for the Southeast Asian region, based in Jakarta, Indonesia. These experiences highlight the sharply contrasting differences in the attitude and aptitude of nutrition students from Asia and Latin America.

Each of the teaching experiences outlined above was associated with collaborative research. This included nickel absorption in Sao Paulo, young child growth in Rio, and urban nutrition of the elderly in Jakarta. The latter is part of a consortium including equivalent research protocols in Mexico and Brazil in this hemisphere and in China, Indonesia, Malaysia, the Philippines, and Thailand in Asia.

What can be construed as my professional activism in Guatemala did not emerge for a decade. Because of the richness and complexity of my chosen second home, I attribute this to the time necessary to assimilate enough of the culture to really function. It also coincides with the end of my "commuter" existence between Cambridge and Guatemala City. Activism in a *professional* sense begins about here in the chronological narrative. Its pursuit fulfills both a dream and an aspiration, namely, that of quality science, reflecting my desire to find solutions to the problems of developing countries, and that of academic freedom, reflecting my desire to train local professionals to be world-class academics.

INCAP in the early 1980s began combining technical assistance with research, to the severe detriment of the research enterprise. Oscar Pineda, a biochemist, intellectual, and visionary, was also disaffected with the sad state of inquiry into which the Institute had fallen. Together, we set about developing a new institution with an old motif. The old motif was fundamental science, driven by hypotheses and crafted by hermetic experimental design. The vehicle, to the extent possible in an impoverished nation, was to be advanced concepts in biology and epidemiology. The Center for Studies of Sensory Impairment, Aging and Metabolism (CeS-SIAM) (in Spanish, *el Centro de Estudios en Sensoriopatias, Senectud e Impedimentos y Alteraciones Metabolicas*) was founded as the research unit for the National Committee for the Blind and Deaf of Guatemala on July 1, 1995. Coming in the month of July, this represented *my* independence day. Doña Elisa Molina de Stahl, the president of the Committee, is a true, authentic Guatemalan activist, a woman who battled all and any odds to bring dignity and resources to the sightless and deaf among the poor. The efficiently and honestly run Committee, a private *patronato,* built a modern eye and ear hospital in 1975. It was into a classroom area of that building that we moved the idea that was CeSSIAM.

We have done good science over the past 10 years. The mission of CeSSIAM is principle driven: quality science and academic freedom. But other principles have emerged, those of opportunity and empowerment. Feminism is only emerging in a Latin context. CeSSIAM was an opportunity to allow women professionals, still blocked from ascent in the domain of clinical medicine, to excel in research. Seventy percent of our professionals have been women; in addition, those of humble families and of indigenous origin have found a door that unlocks new power. My years in Guatemala allowed me to learn enough of the language and culture to undertake building an institution; my sensibilities prompted me to act on "radical" notions such as affirmative opportunities for women and the absence of nepotistic premises. Perhaps these efforts do represent a bit of an expatriate upsetting of the cultural apple cart.

Very recently, I was ever so far away from the East Coast of the United States, yet I did not feel my usual detachment. Rather, I felt connected and yearned to be there! This was on August 28, 1993. I found myself before a cable television on the Island of Bali in Indonesia, taking a few days of "rest" after having finished a brief tour of duty as a consultant and guest faculty member at a Jakarta nutrition program; I was, at the same time, on my way to Melbourne to attend to editing the book, *Dietary Habits in Later Life: A Cross-Cultural Approach.* On the terrace of the Meslati Hotel, I watched a broadcast of the 30th anniversary celebration of the March on Washington for Jobs and Freedom of 1963. Why was I so far away? Why had I not even known it was scheduled? In the old black-and-white newsreel films, I strained to see the spot where the 19-year-old Harvard College freshman had marched behind Bill Russell, Tom Atkins, Ruth Batson, and the Boston NAACP delegation, where he had listened in person to Martin Luther King's "I Have a Dream" oration. Had I been anywhere in the Western Hemisphere that day, I know I would have found a way once again to be beside the Reflecting Pool at the foot of the Lincoln Memorial.

The archive films of the first march revealed so much to me about my innocence, and my lost innocence. Racial equality, not "black power," was the Congress on Racial Equality's shared goal. No one eschewed the use of the word "Negro"; Dr. King, himself, had said, "In the words of the old Negro Spiritual . . . Free at last! Free at last! Thank God Almighty, we're free at last!" As I watched, I reattached myself to my feeling of optimism during that era. Perhaps as a result of beginning to write this chapter (my nerve endings newly enlivened to activism) and in the wake of the XV International Congress on Nutrition, I find myself drawn to professional activism on an even wider (geographically) stage. This may be termed the "last crusade." My travel schedule and development of professional contacts on each of the continents has enabled this new departure. Empowering researchers in nutrition and biomedicine throughout the Third World underlies the three prongs of my post-Adelaide activism. My tool is the pen (or word-processing software) as I am moved to write essays and editorials.

Lately, I have found myself defending the very field I work in. The first salvo in one such skirmish was fired by Alan Berg of the World Bank. He is author of *The Nutrition Factor,* an enlightened call for the inclusion of nutritional concerns in strategies of economic development. His memorial lecture entitled "Sliding toward Nutritional Malpractice: Time to Reconsider and Redeploy" critiqued the focus and priorities of the academic nutrition community in the developing world and called for the creation of a new, applied professional called "nutritional engineers." This suggestion was met by a barrage of letters to the editor from investigators, including me. The discussion began to polarize, and open name-calling between biologists and public health workers in nutrition ensued. From my point of view, inquiry continues to contribute vital new insights into the way that diet, environment, and human metabolism interact. I also believe that serious and detrimental errors can be made by ignoring or misinterpreting valid scientific information. So the editorial activism in me comes forth to defend the legitimacy and value of nutrition research.

Not only should there be research on nutritional problems affecting Third World populations, but it should be second to none in terms of quality and creativity. The second level of activism is to bring *advanced* biology to the service of progress in health and nutrition. Stable isotopes, advanced mathematics of biostatistics and epidemiology, molecular biology techniques, and biotechnology all have the potential to be powerful tools for understanding nutritional problems and their solutions. They also hone the minds of those who use them and impart credibility. Third World nutritional scientists merit access to these modern tools; I am actively devising ways to connect the technologies of the North with inquiry in the South.

Finally, a geographically neutral term for nutritionists concerned with the dietary and nutritional problems of Third World countries needs to be coined. The current term is "international nutrition," a euphemism for nutrition in developing countries or Third World nutrition, both of which have derogatory connotations. But there is a First-World-centric connotation in the use of international, which applies also to public health schools' departments of "International Health." Perhaps "tropical and geographic" nutrition would be more sensitive, more descriptive, and more empowering for those participating from the developing nations, themselves.

SYNTHESIS

In synthesis — and with detachment — I must conclude that my activism has been a species of reactivism. It has not evolved from an adoption of a set of ideological principles chosen on a clear, cerebral basis and embraced with a heartfelt passion. Rather, it has evolved in reaction to circumstances related to race, my perception of racism, and my desire to avoid the personal pain and confusion of racism. It led me to the culture of activism in my student and physician phases and to my expatriate refuge during my professional years. I have lived the activism with passion, but more the passion of a quest than that of conviction. My participation in action for social change was marked by race and North American racism, educated by the thinking and writing of other persons, and sensitized to situations of disadvantaged classes such as the poor, women, Hispanics, Native Americans, and homosexuals. The political currents in the 1960s and 1970s and the professional currents in the 1980s and 1990s added substance, texture, and opportunity. The educational and career choices and the people along the way have provided depth and dimension to the specific activities of my life, both those that are activism and those that are merely action.

To paraphrase an old canon: some people are born activists, some people achieve activism, and others have activism thrust upon them. What has made me an activist has been none of the above but rather a struggle for psychic comfort. The path of least resistance became the choice to resist, to resist the realities and assumptions of racism, resist the injustices committed at home and abroad by U.S. governmental action and inaction, and now to resist mediocrity, irrelevance, and discrimination in science as it develops in Third World countries. My brand of social activism could be regarded as being narrowly conceived, because scientists are those being empowered. But, I hope that unfettered researchers will, through the fruits of their research, lead to further well-being for the less privileged 80% of the world's population.

As a final note, I think of the policy debate taking place over U.S. health care. Rather on CBS and Brokaw on NBC frame the terms of the health care crisis and its resolution, sandwiched between news of another drive-by tourist shooting in Florida and the Major League baseball strike. Across the gulf that separates me from the terms of their debate, the scene stimulates in me paradigms of "healing versus knowing," or "healing through knowing," or "knowing through healing." In writing this book, and in responding to this issue, I realize that I am a physician, an *activist* physician, and a teaching academic, an *activist* academic, and I have finally finished the sharing only to become aware of how much more there is for both you and me to bring forth and analyze.

POSTSCRIPT

Dr. Noel Solomons continues his efforts to shape CeS-SIAM into a self-sustained institution that attracts young scientists and world-class areas of research. Dr. Solomons is editing a book entitled *Child Nutrition: An International Perspective* and has just reconstituted the Committee on Urbanization and Nutrition of the International Union of Nutritional Sciences. He spoke on the subject "Building a Constituency for Nutrition Research in Developing Countries: The Agony and the Ecstacy" at Harvard Medical School's Class of 1970 Twenty-Fifth Reunion in Boston. His upcoming foreign lecturing and travel plans include the United States, Indonesia, China, and Peru.

CHAPTER VIII

IMPROVING AMERICAN INDIAN HEALTH

EDITH R. WELTY, M.D. and, THOMAS K. WELTY, M.D., M.P.H.

In this autobiographical chapter, we have focused on the parts of our lives most likely to provide a unique perspective for health care professionals. By describing certain types of personal and professional experiences, we aim to encourage and inform medical students and physicians interested in social change. For those in the medical profession, we hope that our stories will stimulate some of you to seek innovative ways to identify and prioritize health problems and to improve medical care. In the hopes that readers may benefit, we have included not only successes but mistakes. We have never perceived our work as requiring major sacrifices. On the contrary, we have enjoyed the cross-cultural relationships with American Indians, the challenge and gratification of helping to improve medical care on a community-wide basis, and the outdoor life-style afforded by the rural locations where we have lived. We have chosen to write in the third person to enable us to express ourselves as individuals rather than as a unit.

CHILDHOOD EXPERIENCES

Edie was on born October 9, 1942 to John and Ruth Roberts in New Kensington, Pennsylvania, a steel mill town on the Allegheny River. John was a steel worker who spent his entire career working for the Allegheny Ludlum Corporation, retiring after 42 years of service. Edie's father was always fair and evenhanded in his dealings with others regardless of their social status, race, or ethnicity. His work in the steel mill reinforced these tendencies; this leveling ground required all sorts of workers to function as a team under very difficult circumstances. Ruth was a dental hygienist who was also active in the Baptist church. When Edie, the youngest of three children, was growing up, Ruth was a full-time mom. The Roberts family valued education, and all three siblings ended up with college or higher degrees. Despite their differing beliefs (John was an agnostic), John and Ruth's relationship was based on love and respect and lasted for over 50 years until John's death in 1986.

Edie's parents combined support of activities they approved of with flexibility and tolerance regarding others. For example, in addition to encouraging her academic achievements, Edie's parents promoted her competition in diving and gymnastics. On the other hand, the Roberts children routinely attended Baptist Sunday school and church, but John's agnosticism bolstered them when they preferred not to participate. Similarly, Edie's parents patiently stood by as their daughter became fervently attached to an Evangelical fundamentalist sect, ultimately joining the Youth for Christ movement. These flashes of independence, competitive experiences, and the discipline of athletic training provided Edie with the tenacity required to flourish in medical school, as a mother, and as a doctor.

Edie's college years proved to be transformative ones in which she began to discover the values that would sustain her over the course of her career. Initially, Edie's fundamental Christian beliefs led her to attend Wheaton College, a Fundamentalist Christian college in Wheaton, Illinois. An anthropology course at this college stimulated Edie to question her beliefs and to learn the tenets of other faiths. After two years, she transferred to Penn State, which was closer to her home, less expensive, and more in tune with her evolving beliefs. Increasingly, Edie's goals were based on social consciousness rather than the dictates of religious persuasion. For example, Edie's initial motivation to pursue medicine was to serve as a medical missionary in Africa, an ambition replaced by a more general desire to serve disadvantaged peoples.

Tom was born November 7, 1943 in Homestead, Pennsylvania. Tom's father, Fred, served as the minister of music at a Presbyterian Church, and his mother, Margaret, served as the organist. Theirs was a happy marriage in which life's pleasures and sorrows were shared on both a personal and professional level. Fred and Margaret worked closely with each other in their chosen field of religious music and also supported each other in gardening and Christmas tree farming. Tom was born when Margaret was 39 years old, after 13 years of marriage.

The notion of a Christmas tree farm grew out of Fred and Margaret's 1950 purchase of 79 acres of overgrown western Pennsylvania farmland, appropriately named Welty's Windy Wilderness. Through the next 15 years Tom's parents devoted prodigious energy to converting the wilderness to Welty's Wooded Wonderland. This land provided an excellent escape from church politics, was a unifying force in the family, and eventually yielded acres and acres of Christmas trees. Fred and Margaret also cultivated a garden each year to help supplement the family's modest income. Because of all these activities, and because of the family's frugal ethos, there always seemed to be sufficient funds to support the family. Tom absorbed his parents' thrifty ways; for example, from age 10 through high school, Tom sold garden produce door to door from a Red Flier wagon. Because of his success in this venture, he saved enough money to buy a 1950 GMC pickup truck in 1959 at age 16. This pickup truck served him well through high school, college, and medical school. It was replaced only when its failing health raised doubts that it would get Edie to the hospital when she went into labor.

As a PK (preacher's kid), and as a "normal" adolescent, it was important for Tom to "act out" in some way. He accomplished this by totally rejecting all aspects of music. During these rebellious years, Tom hid the piano books during lessons and refused to sing when participating in choir performances. Although Tom never learned to read music or to play an instrument, he later softened and sang in high school and college choirs. During Tom's college years, his Presbyterian upbringing had a somewhat different effect, resulting in an inclination toward a career in the ministry. Similarly to Edie, however, his beliefs in the Presbyterian dogma gradually shifted toward those of an agnostic. His career goals newly oriented, Tom's commitment to providing altruistic service remained steadfast throughout his professional career.

As Tom considered which college to attend, the College of Wooster in Wooster, Ohio seemed logical. This college provided an excellent liberal arts curriculum, had a good premedical program, and was affiliated with the Presbyterian church, and Tom had family members on both sides who had graduated from the institution. As an undergraduate, the rigors of the chemistry department prepared Tom well for the challenges of medical school, and a summer study program in Vienna broadened his horizons and enabled him to become fluent in German. The summer of 1964 was a critical time for Tom's decision to go into medicine: he worked and observed at the Radiology Department at Latrobe Hospital under the supervision of Dr. Francis Feightner, the father of his best friend. That summer was also critical in gaining practical skills, as Tom contributed to all aspects of constructing his parents' new house.

After graduating in 1965, Tom spent the summer at the Beacon Neighborhood House in Chicago conducting an educational enrichment program for African-American youths. The experience of sharing a three-room tenement with seven co-workers in the black ghetto and witnessing inner-city life first hand furthered Tom's commitment to social justice. Hearing Martin Luther King's addresses — one in particular was directed toward residents of Chicago tenements — powerfully reinforced Tom's growing idealism. One of the happiest moments of Tom's young life was in August, 1965, when his parents visited him in Chicago. They brought a huge garbage can filled with fresh sweet corn from the garden and prepared a neighborhood picnic that was thoroughly enjoyed by the African-American community.

Two weeks later tragedy struck. Tom returned home to find his father hospitalized after having collapsed while chopping down a large tree. His father seemed to be on the road to recovery but died suddenly on August 20, 1965 as the result of a highly unusual condition, the rupture of a pulmonary aneurysm. It seemed that the decision to go to Pittsburgh Medical School was predestined, because Tom's proximity to his mother allowed him to provide support during the grieving process. Together they weathered this transition, and Margaret decided she could remain at her newly completed home.

MEDICAL SCHOOL

Tom and Edie met during their junior (Edie's) and sophomore (Tom's) years at Pittsburgh School of Medicine, a meeting that culminated in a romance, engagement, and marriage lasting more than 25 years. Their enduring partnership is based on mutual respect, professional cooperation, and a love that has grown stronger through the years. Theirs was not a love at first sight but one that developed gradually as they realized the many values they held in common.

Tom and Edie's reactions to medical school differed considerably, possibly because of the divergent attitudes of their respective classes. Overall, Tom's class (1969) was altruistically motivated and characterized the spirit of the 1960s, whereas Edie's class (1968) was competitive and seemed to be largely motivated by mercenary goals. Edie's first 2 years were stressful, as a result of her own exceptionally high standards and her status as one of only six women in the class. She struggled through biochemistry and physiology and nearly gave up after panicking during her first few internal medicine case presentations. The hands-on patient care of the third and fourth years was much more to her liking, and she passed these years with flying colors.

Through the Christian Medical Society, Tom met Edie and began borrowing things such as her embryology book, microscope, and other useful items that were no longer needed by the upper class. In the summer of 1966, both worked with Dr. Francis Drew and Dr. Ken Rogers on a community medicine externship. Edie's project that summer was to measure blood pressures in male black adolescents in a Pittsburgh housing project. Tom, after working on his own project, was assigned to Edie's to serve as a stern-appearing control: because the blood pressures obtained by Edie were lower than blood pressures obtained for black children in other studies, fellow externs thought that Edie's laid-back approach accounted for the discrepancy. (This theory was not confirmed; Tom's results were similar to Edie's.)[1]

The following summer Tom bought a 1956 VW bus at an auction. Accompanied by a classmate, he set off for the wilds of the Navajo reservation in Arizona to do community medicine projects. He loaned his 1950 GMC truck to Edie for the summer because she had to remain in Pittsburgh to repeat her internal medicine rotation. At the end of the summer, Edie came to Arizona where, amid the lovely Chuska Mountains, she became engaged to Tom with marriage planned in April 1968. This summer was instrumental to Tom and Edie's professional life as well as their personal one. Tom's positive experience in Indian Health Service, as well as the possibility of fulfilling his draft obligations, eventually attracted them back to IHS.

MARRIAGE AND POSTGRADUATE TRAINING

Over the next few months, Tom and Edie orchestrated a rapid succession of events. Their wedding was on April 15, 1968, immediately after Edie's senior class play (for which she was Master of Ceremonies) and 6 weeks before her graduation. The bride prepared most of the food for a reception for 150 people and was a few minutes late because she was frantically putting last-minute hors d'oeuvres in the oven. A few days after the honeymoon in Miami Beach, Edie took her National Board exams. Needless to say, she did not study very hard for them.

Their first child, Julie, was born in October 1969 at Mercy Hospital in Pittsburgh, where Edie was in an internal medicine residency and Tom was in a rotating internship. Ironically, Edie was Tom's resident at the time of Julie's birth. To obtain care for their newborn, they requested and received permission from Mercy's administration to keep Julie in a seldom-used premature isolation nursery. The nurses were delighted to have a healthy baby to play with, and Edie was able to breast-feed while on call every third or fourth night. When Edie's pager beeped, it meant either an emergency in intensive care or Julie was hungry.

Tom and Edie were pleased with the postgraduate training they received at Mercy Hospital, in terms of both its depth and scope of training and its commitment to disadvantaged populations. Because this hospital was Pittsburgh's primary facility providing care to poor patients, house staff saw a wide range of clinical problems, trauma, and serious social problems. This exposure served Tom and Edie well in preparation for work with the Indian Health Service. It was indeed a privilege to work in an institution dedicated to meeting the health needs of its community, regardless of ability to pay, and to responding to the parenting needs of house staff.

RECRUITMENT AND RETENTION WITH THE INDIAN HEALTH SERVICE

After their tenure at Mercy Hospital, Tom and Edie embarked on their assignment with IHS in Tuba City, Arizona. The IHS fulfilled Tom's draft obligation, seemed a much more attractive alternative than Vietnam, and required only a 2-year commitment. Tom, Edie (4 months pregnant), daughter Julie, and Tom's mother Margaret arrived in Tuba City in the midst of a sandstorm. When they saw their assigned house, with sand sifting in through ill-fitting windows, they felt they would be lucky to survive there for 2 years.

However, a number of factors kept Tom and Edie in Arizona for 12 years. First, after living in a small apartment in Pittsburgh, the three-bedroom government house — aside from the recurring red sand — seemed palatial. Second, child care arrangements were the best possible for parents who both worked well over 40 hours per week.

These child care arrangements fell into place largely by chance. During their first week in Tuba City, Tom and Edie were approached by a Hopi couple, Russell and Virginia Gaseoma, who offered to provide child care for Julie. Virginia had eight children of her own, the youngest of whom was 4 years old, and Russell worked as a bus driver. This couple proved to be enormously important to the Weltys, by providing tangible support and a vital link to the Indian community. With child care arrangements finalized and Tom's mother back in Pennsylvania, Tom and Edie launched their careers with the Indian Health Service.

Edie remained extremely active during her pregnancy, including riding to the Keetseel ruins on horseback and taking a 3-day raft trip and hike in the Grand Canyon. These were activities that perhaps were not advisable at 7 months of gestation, especially because the horseback ride initiated a burst of premature contractions. Edie chose to have Anna at home with only Tom attending because some hospital personnel frowned on the presence of family members at childbirth. To prepare for childbirth, Edie spread a large plastic sheet on the bed, placed Julie (then 14 months old) in her crib with the phone book to tear up for entertainment, set up two chairs for foot support, and showered. Tom arrived home with the delivery pack just as Anna's head emerged, and was met with vigorous cries from his new daughter. This occurred on December 16, 1970, 2 hours after Edie completed a full day in clinic. A few hours later, Edie and Tom made a brief appearance at a Christmas party. After taking 1 week off from work, Edie went back to her full time duties.

Tom and Edie's relationship with Virginia and Russell was mutually beneficial and encompassed more than "professional" responsibilities. For example, the Indian couple had been married in the traditional Hopi way for many years but had never legally declared their marriage. Russell was a World War II veteran, and lack of legal marriage meant that Virginia would not be eligible for benefits available to spouses of veterans. Tom and Edie helped them marry according to United States laws, made a cake, and hosted a ceremony.

Tom and Edie encouraged their children to become immersed in Hopi life, and Virginia seemed to welcome the opportunity to share her culture. She often took the children to the Hopi village where they participated in day-to-day activities with the Hopi children (e.g., hauling water from the village well). On those days the children were exposed to various aspects of Hopi life, learned some of the language, and received the names of Saquapu (blue corn) and Digoodie (yellow corn).

Thus, the children spent their formative years as a racial minority deeply enmeshed in a mixture of cultures. Although Julie and Anna experienced racial prejudice on a number of occasions, the experience of growing up on the Navajo Reservation was a positive one overall. The environment was stimulating throughout their childhood years and fostered self-esteem and a fairness that overcame prejudice.

The recreational activities in the Four Corners area were a major factor in the Weltys' decision to stay in Tuba City. On every free weekend, they would hop into their four-wheel drive International Travelall, affectionately named Big Red, and explore the reservation's remote regions as well as parks and national monuments. When the girls were less than 3 years old, the family hiked from Coal Mine Canyon down Moencopi Wash and 20 miles back to Tuba City (Mom and Dad carried them most of the way). At least once a year, Edie and Tom would take a long backpack through the Grand Canyon or another isolated area, leaving the kids with the Gaseomas.

During the 12 years they spent in Tuba City, the Welty's association with a foster child was one of their most troubling experiences. In retrospect, this child's behavior was characteristic of that associated with fetal alcohol exposure, as described by Michael Dorris in his book *The Broken Cord*.[2] It was very difficult to understand her behavior, and, most importantly, to help her establish acceptable social relationships. This child's plight made clear the disastrous social, medical, and economic consequences of fetal alcohol exposure and became the stimulus for Tom later to develop screening strategies for FAS.[3]

TOM'S GROWING INTEREST IN PUBLIC HEALTH
AND INTERNATIONAL HEALTH

During medical school Tom made several international trips with the Brother's Brother Foundation, a private, non-profit foundation. For Tom, these trips underscored medicine's capacity to dramatically improve public health while also showing the ruthless role of economics in determining each individual's fate. Working in Central America, Tom and foundation personnel provided donated vaccine and technical assistance to implement mass immunization programs. Tom worked under the direction of Dr. Robert Hingson, who invented the jet injector gun — at the time the best way to provide mass immunizations in developing countries. As a consequence of these early exposures to public health and international health, Tom subsequently worked on the following projects:

1. The Bolivian Campaign (1969). Shortly after Julie was born, Dr. Hingson invited Tom and Edie to participate in a mass immunization program in La Paz, Bolivia. While her parents were immunizing, Julie was cared for by missionaries in La Paz. She was the only family member who had no adverse effects from altitude sickness (La Paz is 12,000 feet above sea level) or Montezuma's revenge (because she was breast-feeding). As part of a large public health team, Tom and Edie had a wonderful experience providing smallpox, measles, BCG, and DPT to a total of 180,000 individuals during this 2-week period. This was accomplished by coordinating the public health department, volunteers from Brother's Brother Foundation, and the Bolivian military.

2. Haiti (1972). Dr. Hingson invited Tom to be the project coordinator for a Haitian immunization program designed to provide three DPT and polio immuniza-

tions. Working with a team from the Ministry of Health, Brother's Brother immunized many isolated communities in the region of Thomaseau. The abject poverty and inadequacies of both public health and primary care were appalling and led Tom to a much greater appreciation of the level of health care provided by the Indian Health Service. Two vivid experiences illustrate the deprivation of the Haitian people. First, a mother offered Tom a meager sum to take her child with him back to the United States. Second, Tom witnessed the plight of children hospitalized at the University Hospital, where no medications were available unless the young patients' impoverished parents paid for the drugs. Frequently children with pneumonia or other treatable infections would die for lack of antibiotics. Because of time constraints, the overworked nurses would wait for several children to die before they transported the bodies to the morgue.

3. China. Tom accompanied Dr. Hingson to China in 1980 to demonstrate the jet injectors to the Chinese Ministry of Health. This visit was conducted in conjunction with American orthopedic surgeons, who were learning about Chinese orthopedic techniques. China had only recently opened to the West, and the Chinese were eager for as much interchange as possible. He observed a Chinese woman having a cesarean section under acupuncture anesthesia, Chinese orthopedic techniques, and health care delivery on a commune and in several urban settings.

Tom was inspired by China's public health approach toward its massive medical problems.[4] For example, he heard Dr. George Hatem (Dr. Ma Hai-Teh) describe how sexually transmitted diseases (STDs) were eliminated by the Mao Zedong regime after the "Long March." Dr. Hatem, a Lebanese-American physician, recruited Chinese prostitutes as STD control workers, and after appropriate treatment, STDs gradually disappeared. The communists also promoted equality of women and the concept of one child per family, both of which were critically important for social, political, economic, and health reasons.

The generosity of the Chinese was overwhelming. They gave multiple banquets and beautiful gifts to the Americans in appreciation for the jet injectors and technical advice. Two of the Chinese surgeons who served as guides for the 2 weeks visited Tom and Edie in Tuba City in 1981 and 1982. They both enjoyed making home visits to Navajo and Hopi families and stated that the pueblos were very similar to villages in Tibet.

THE MEDICAL EXPERIENCE IN TUBA CITY

In Tuba City, Tom and Edie worked under the only surgeon at this 75-bed facility and were expected to perform all aspects of clinical services. Tom became Director of Community Health Services, and Edie worked in a full-time clinical capacity rotating on Pediatrics, Internal Medicine, Obstetrics, and Surgery as well as in the Outpatient Department. Initially there was no board-certified internist at Tuba City, and so she served as the chief of medicine for the first 2 years. Because of staff shortages at the clinic, Tom and Edie were often required to adopt multiple roles.

Although the specialty of Family Practice did not exist at the time Tom and Edie began their careers in IHS, the clinical experiences at Tuba City resembled current family practice residency programs. Under a "grandfather clause" for those already in practice prior to the establishment of family practice residencies, Tom and Edie were eligible to take family practice boards in 1974 and thereby became Diplomates of the newly established American Board of Family Practice.

In Tuba City, Tom and Edie experienced both the fulfillment of practicing medicine, and the frustrations of inadequate funding. American Indians and Alaska Natives, are eligible for services similar to those provided by a prepaid health maintenance organization combined with a public health department. Thus, IHS clinical services are much more closely integrated with preventive and community health services than in other segments of the United States. For example, one of the innovative approaches to ambulatory care IHS advocates is "industrial strength triage." This concept emphasizes the need to systematically review patient charts and provide preventive services to all patients, regardless of the chief complaint that brought them to the hospital or clinic.

However, the approach to medical care in the Indian Health Service is hampered by insufficient funding, and rationing of medical care is standard practice. In larger IHS hospitals, such as Tuba City, elective surgical procedures are provided with minimal delays. However, in more remote facilities, surgical and other specialty services sometimes are not available. Even in Tuba City, the outpatient department had a woefully small number of examining rooms, and these were not sufficiently private. In the early 1970s, Tom and Edie helped justify and plan a new facility, which received federal funding. Eventually a new 100-bed hospital was completed, including a larger outpatient department, increased staff, and more space.

In addition to contending with IHS's systemic problems, the Weltys' day-to-day practice presented unique challenges. About half of Tom and Edie's adult patients spoke no English. Although the Weltys learned enough Navajo to perform a physical exam and take superficial histories, interpreters were required for in-depth communication.

Traditional Navajo beliefs had a significant impact on Tom and Edie's patients. In one case, a young woman who was 7 months pregnant was brought to the hospital unconscious following several seizures at home. She had had a normal exam in the prenatal clinic the previous week. Although Edie maintained her on a respirator, induced labor, and controlled her hypertension, the woman died the next day. According to her family, the woman had been well until she saw a "skinwalker" (werewolf) outside her hogan. According to Navajo tradition, evil people sometimes dress up as skinwalkers to carry out witchcraft, and their curses can be deadly. Or, Edie wondered, was this just a case of eclampsia with disseminated intravascular coagulation or a ruptured cerebral aneurysm?

Another example of witchcraft was the case of a high school senior who accidentally burned down a house with gas fumes from his motorcycle, killing his aunt and nephew. Edie treated this young man for minor burns and smoke inhalation. Initially, he seemed minimally ill. His family, however, blamed him for the deaths and hired a Navajo herbalist. After each visit from the herbalist, the man took a turn for the worse. Relatives told him that they saw ravens flying through the roof of the burned house and that he must die. Although all laboratory and X-ray findings were normal, the young man had a sudden respiratory arrest while talking with the psychiatrist. Edie intubated him and put him on a respirator. The boy gradually died in "perfect chemical balance." Funeral plans, plus warnings not to interfere with traditional practices, persuaded the Service Unit Director to direct Edie not to push for an autopsy. Thus, the boy apparently succumbed to either a "voodoo death" of sorts or else herbal poisons.

Skinwalkers and witches represent only the dark side of Navajo traditions. On the other side of the coin are the traditional healers who undo evil, usually through "Sings" or chants that can vary in length from hours to days. There are also "crystal gazers" (diagnosticians) and healing herbalists.

On one occasion an elderly man who had a brainstem stroke was deteriorating and unable to swallow and was being nourished in the hospital through a nasogastric tube. The family brought in a medicine man who, with the internist's permission, diluted an herbal remedy and squirted it down the tube with a syringe. The patient immediately improved and was able to go home a few days later.

On another occasion, a medicine man approached Tom about a mutual patient. The medicine man had diagnosed the old lady as having pneumonia, performed a healing ceremony, and then recommended that she go to the hospital. The old lady had refused, presumably because she lived far out in a canyon and had her 12-year-old granddaughter living with her (truant from school). Tom saw the woman in clinic and confirmed the medicine man's diagnosis, but neither could persuade her to be hospitalized. Tom gave her intramuscular and oral penicillin and arranged for daily visits by the public health nurse, and the patient recovered.

Medicine men often performed short ceremonies and then referred patients to the hospital, illustrating the cooperation that occurred between traditional and modern healers. For example, some medicine men would "suck" gallstones from patients, but if symptoms continued, the afflicted individuals would come to IHS for removal of the one last stone missed by the healer. At times sick children would arrive at the hospital covered with charcoal from a ceremony, and the parents would request IV hydration. Dr. Jean Van Duzen, a career IHS pediatrician, remembers the occasion when a family walked many miles carrying a dead baby to the hospital because they had heard that she could bring babies back to life with IV therapy.

The more culturally sensitive IHS physicians also referred appropriate patients to traditional healers. Despite the intricacies of this type of referral, Tom and Edie felt it was required in order to heal certain patients. Proper referral required understanding about the beliefs of the patient's family and the appropriate traditional treatment for a given disease. One had to know whether the family used traditional Navajo medicine men, Native American Church (peyote religion), Christianity, or a combination of all of these.

If, for example, a Vietnam vet from a traditional Navajo family was having psychiatric disturbances, he might need an Enemy Way Sing to remove the ghost of a dead person he had seen (seeing dead people is taboo) before psychotherapy or medication would help him. Because the patient himself could not request a Sing, one must politely suggest a ceremony to the appropriate family member. Some Sings were very expensive for the family, requiring them to put on a feast for many relatives in addition to paying the medicine man. Other Sings called for special hogans and sand paintings, for which medicine men gathered properly colored sand from remote locations.

Perhaps the funniest tale of patient care involved a pregnant woman who had broken her leg. She lived a few miles out on a dirt road from Tom's field clinic in Kaibeto. The woman's relatives worried that she might go into labor while trapped at home with a cast on her leg, so they asked Tom to make a home visit. The road had recently been washed out by heavy rains, so Tom and the driver/interpreter began walking through the mud toward the woman's home. When the driver/interpreter saw a horse tied outside the trading post, he suggested they ride. They mounted the horse, made the home visit, and were assured by the woman that she was not in labor. Upon their return, the horse's owner spied them just when they came over the hill to the trading post. The driver/interpreter jumped off, leaving Tom riding in as the guilty horse thief.

In 1972, Edie became the director of the outpatient department and became more involved in the obstetric service. Many of the pregnant teenagers sought her services because they preferred to see a woman doctor; their large numbers led her to study the rates of teenage pregnancy in the public schools. She found that about a third of the high school seniors and a fourth of the juniors either were pregnant or had been pregnant. Over the course of the next 5 years, she made intensive efforts to persuade the community and the schools to institute a sex education program. Shortly after she succeeded, the *Navajo Times* acquired a copy of her teen pregnancy study and published an article on the high pregnancy rates in Tuba City schools. School officials were so offended that they not only discontinued the sex ed program but would not even allow dental hygienists to lecture to students. This was quite a lesson in how efforts at social change can backfire if press coverage seems to cast a negative image of the community.

As Director of Community Health, Tom supervised public health nurses, several driver/interpreters, and TB and maternal/child health workers. He was responsible for providing clinical services to outlying field clinics, which were 30–60 miles from the Tuba City Hospital. These field clinics, held once or twice a week, provided well-child care, prenatal care, and follow-up of chronic diseases. Tom developed strategies to combat the Navajos' major health problems, including problems brought on or exacerbated by the poverty of reservation life and flawed government policies.

At that time, the major health problems of the Navajos still were infectious diseases and malnutrition. Before the synthesis of isoniazid (INH), patients were treated in sanatoria hundreds of miles from their homes for months or years and sometimes until their deaths. In the late 1960s, IHS wisely began emphasizing INH prophylaxis of tuberculin reactors, and Indian TB rates decreased among American Indians and Alaska Natives more rapidly than the national rates. In the late 1970s, the standard of care for treatment of active TB became supervised, directly observed, twice-weekly therapy after an initial 2-month period of daily therapy. Tom treated about 50 patients with active TB and dispensed prophylaxis to hundreds of TB reactors, converters, and contacts. This experience enabled him to develop standards of care for treatment of TB in IHS,[5,6] and further study confirmed the benefits of INH chemoprophylaxis in Oglala Sioux Indian patients.[7]

Malnutrition was a major contributor to the high rates of infectious diseases afflicting Indian children. In the late 1960s, there was extensive discussion as to whether Indian children should be assigned different growth curves from the national norms, as so many were small.[8] Dr. Jean VanDuzen, a pediatrician who spent her entire career in Tuba City, documented the malnutrition that afflicted Indian children, including cases of kwashiorkor and marasmus.[9] As a result of her efforts and other reports of malnutrition among American Indians and Alaska Natives, extensive feeding programs were implemented, including commodity foods, formula programs for infants, WIC, and food stamps. In the space of one generation, these programs virtually eliminated malnutrition.

Now Indian children generally exceed the national growth curves. The high fat and low fiber content of foods provided to these people through the commodities program accelerated the development of obesity and its complications. There is again discussion about creating separate growth curves for Indian children, because they are so heavy. The problems of obesity, smoking, diabetes, coronary heart disease, hypertension, and cancer have replaced the problems of malnutrition and infectious diseases as leading health concerns for Indian people during the 1980s and 1990s.[10,11]

The government response to the reservation's sanitation problems was, like the commodities program, well-intentioned with similarly unfortunate effects. Initially, the government envisioned the continuance of rural life-styles by providing wells pumped by windmills. However, in the early 1970s, Navajo families lived in isolated camps many miles from paved roads and frequently had to haul water 10 or 20 miles. This resulted in inadequate supplies of water for washing and often in contaminated drinking water. Infantile diarrhea, particularly shigellosis, became epidemic during the summer and fall months.[12,13] Malnourished children became critically ill when infected with shigellosis and other enteric pathogens.

Funding was appropriated through Congress to provide water and sewage systems for Indian homes. In order to comply with new regulations, "cluster housing" was planned and built, with support from the Department of Housing and Urban Development. Although the program was quite successful in reducing the rates of enteric illness and the rates of infant death from complications of enteric disease, it introduced a whole new set of social problems. Traditional families were forced to give up their subsistence life-styles, based on herding sheep and farming, to move into cluster homes. High unemployment rates, alcohol abuse, and a sedentary life-style led to new problems with increasing rates of chronic disease.[11]

In addition to attending to the structural and systemic problems affecting American Indians and Alaska Natives, Tom also focused on treating their resultant medical problems. He mobilized resources to combat middle ear disease, trachoma, and several cases of plague among these people. Among Navajo children at that time, middle ear disease, particularly eardrum perforation, was rampant. Because there was no ENT specialist available, Tom implemented a program that brought in ENT specialists from the University of Pittsburgh. These physicians performed over 100 tympanoplasties, thus eliminating the backlog of children with perforated eardrums who had heretofore been unable to obtain the recommended surgery because of the limited staff and resources in IHS.[14] Trachoma and resulting blindness were also serious health problems among Indians of the Southwest; through a program of systematic screening and treatment and the improvement of hygienic conditions, trachoma was virtually eliminated as a health problem among these people.[15]

Plague (*Yersinia pestis*) occurs more commonly in the Western Navajo than perhaps anywhere else in the country.[16]

In 1976, Edie cared for the first case reported in many years: a pregnant woman from Navajo Mountain who arrived with a high fever of unknown cause. Subsequently, an additional 18 cases of plague were diagnosed and successfully treated at Tuba City.[16–18]

In 1976, Tom was selected as Service Unit Director (SUD) for Tuba City. As the SUD, he was responsible for hospital-based clinical services, Community Health Services, the Environmental Health Program (which, among other tasks, provided water and sewage systems to Indian homes), and for providing and maintaining 200 housing units for hospital employees. To facilitate these activities, he worked closely with the Indian Health Advisory Board, a group of community members that functioned essentially as a Board of Directors for the Service Unit. Tom met with the Board on a regular basis to update them on health problems and new health initiatives and to solicit their input and guidance.

TRANSITION TO CDC

After 12 years in Tuba City, Tom and Edie felt the need for additional training and challenges. They transferred to a 2-year program at the Centers for Disease Control's Epidemic Intelligence Service (EIS) and continued for a third year as preventive medicine residents. Edie worked for 2 years in Special Studies Branch, establishing a protocol for determining whether significant exposure to toxic waste, especially polychlorinated biphenyls (PCBs), had occurred.[19] Subsequently, she spent a year working in the Sexually Transmitted Diseases Division. Tom spent the entire 3 years working in cancer epidemiology.

The transition from the remote desert community of Tuba City to the sprawling urban metropolis of Atlanta was somewhat traumatic to the family, especially to Julie, who had difficulty finding friends. However, professional experiences at CDC broadened Tom's and Edie's outlook on medicine and public health and provided them with skills that would be helpful on return to the Indian Health Service.

In 1984–1985, her third year at CDC, Edie performed quality assurance reviews of STD clinics throughout the nation and lectured to state health departments on the medical epidemiology of AIDS and the new ELISA HIV test. Tom learned how to design and implement large case-control and cohort studies by working on the Agent Orange Study. He also worked on the "Closing the Gap" project, a preventive medicine effort supported by President Carter through Emory University.[20]

While in Atlanta, Tom completed a Masters Degree in Public Health at Emory University. This program was very flexible and compatible with the schedules required of an EIS/preventive medicine resident. His M.P.H. courses, which lasted a year and a half, integrated quite well into the daily work at CDC, and his thesis on the health effects of salty drinking water in Gila Bend, Arizona, gave him a background in cardiovascular disease epidemiology.[21]

RETURN TO THE INDIAN HEALTH SERVICE

The possibility of permanent positions at CDC, although somewhat appealing, did not end the Weltys' yearning to return to the frontier of the American West and the challenges of Indian Health Service. To find a satisfactory site for relocation, Tom and Edie visited Gallup, New Mexico, Phoenix, Tuba City, Anchorage, and Rapid City, North Dakota. The last, the Aberdeen Area Indian Health Service based in Rapid City, seemed to present the greatest professional challenges and was located near natural beauty to boot. (A visit to Rapid City with a tour of the Black Hills and a hike to Harney Peak, the highest peak between the Rockies and the Alps, convinced the Welty family that life in South Dakota would be compatible with their outdoor interests.)

In July 1985, the Welty family moved to Rapid City to seek solutions to the area's severe Indian health problems. As an epidemiologist, Tom found that the health statistics for the Aberdeen Area (which includes North and South Dakota, Nebraska, and Iowa Indians, a total population of 80,000) were the worst of all 12 IHS areas.[22] Infant mortality rates had stabilized at 20 per 1000 live births, with a very high rate of sudden infant death syndrome (SIDS).[23] Mortality rates from chronic diseases, including heart disease, cancer, and diabetes, exceeded rates in all other areas.[24-30] Mortality rates from infectious diseases were decreasing but were still quite high.

Under Tom's supervision, the Aberdeen Area Epidemiology Program grew from a staff of one in 1985 to a multidisciplinary program responsible for communicable disease control, maternal and child health, chronic disease prevention and control, and several research projects. During this time, a number of medical students worked on community medicine projects, developing descriptive data that were very useful for further program development.

Tom also served as the IHS lead epidemiologist on the IHS "Closing the Gap" project (a follow-up of the Carter Center's project) and subsequently published a report entitled *Indian Health Conditions*.[22] This report reviewed 14 major health conditions affecting American Indians and Alaska Natives people and included specific recommendations on how morbidity and mortality rates could be reduced. In addition, Tom worked to adapt existing strategies of providing care to the American Indians and Alaska Natives. For example, Tom helped modify some computer software developed by the Carter Center for "Healthier People HRA" and created a Native American health risk appraisal specific for Native Americans that is now widely available throughout IHS.[31,32]

Just as the couple interacted with community leaders and healers in Tuba City, they developed connections within

Indian communities throughout the area that enabled effective dissemination of health information. For example, in 1988 Tom worked with Colleen Good Bear, the substance abuse coordinator for the Aberdeen Area, and Richard Moves Camp, a traditional Sundance leader, to provide training on preventing the transmission of HIV. As a result, many traditional Sundance leaders take recommended precautions when doing skin piercing, a practice that is part of these sacred ceremonies.

Tom believed the solutions to many of the health problems afflicting Northern Plains Indians lay within the community members themselves. In an effort to empower these people, training entitled "Groundswell toward Health" was provided for community leaders.[33] Training emphasized the benefits of traditional values and beliefs in promoting health at the community level. *Restoring Balance,* a manual outlining how communities can implement preventive health programs, was an outgrowth of this process.[34]

Tom was also involved in multiple efforts to improve care for women, including pregnant women and newborns. For example, he studied how to best provide mammography screening to remote Indian communities, he supported the efforts of the Aberdeen Area Tribal Chairmen's Health Board to obtain a Healthy Start Grant, the only such program targeted toward a Indian population, and he developed an infant mortality case-control study. In addition, he helped obtain a grant funding community response teams for Fetal Alcohol Syndrome (FAS) preventive activities and an FAS and maternal substance abuse surveillance program.

To learn more about cardiovascular disease and its risk factors, Tom applied for and was awarded a 3-year grant to study cardiovascular disease among American Indians. This multicenter study, entitled the "Strong Heart" study, successfully recruited 1500 participants aged 45–75 years and has been funded for a 5-year extension.[35,36]

Edie initially worked as the assistant quality assurance officer and subsequently as physician recruiter for the Aberdeen Area. She greatly preferred clinical medicine and felt unfulfilled when not caring for patients. Thus, in 1987, when the opportunity arose, she gladly resigned from recruiting to start up an ob–gyn program for the Rapid City IHS Hospital (known as "Sioux San" because the facility was initially a TB sanitarium). This program was conceived in response to a crisis in 1985, when many Indian women were left with late or inadequate prenatal and obstetric care. Because no funds were available to construct a birthing center within Sioux San, the service unit initially detailed one physician to acquire privileges to deliver babies at Regional Hospital, the only tertiary care level hospital in a 200-mile radius, and then established a new position for an obstetrician–gynecologist.

Retaining obstetricians at federal salary level is difficult, as this specialty makes three to four times as much in private practice. Thus, as the service unit's ob–gyn patient population was growing by leaps and bounds, their obstetrician was receiving offers from private (nonfederal) groups that, eventually, he could not refuse. In response to this new crisis, the Health Board in 1989 applied to take over the ob–gyn program from IHS so that it would not be limited by federal salaries.[36] This program has been quite successful, as summarized below from an article that was published in the newspaper *Indian County Today* in May 1993.

Health Board up to Something Good with Ob/Gyn Program

Three serious problems in Aberdeen Area are: 1) the high mortality, rates (especially infant mortality which is one of the highest rates in the nation); 2) the lack of a regional IHS referral center; and 3) the severe difficulty of recruiting and retaining physicians, especially in rural service units.

The repeated pattern of physicians leaving due to burnout and the resultant need to use short-term temporary doctors to fill shortages causes loss of continuity in care and limited ability to develop long-range health programs.

With no central referral IHS hospital, each service unit must develop its own referral patterns for patients too ill to be cared for on site to private physicians in a variety of hospitals. With rapid turnover of physicians at the service unit, this becomes confusing and contributes further to loss of continuity of care, physician burnout, and ultimately to higher mortality rates.

This is particularly true for obstetrics, in which health outcomes have been clearly linked to early and adequate prenatal care, and high-risk mothers and babies are more safely delivered in centers with surgical and neonatal capabilities.

The Rapid City Indian Health Board (RCIHB) is in the process of planning to send its OB/GYN Program physicians to provide two clinics plus one night of call each week at Eagle Butte, Rosebud, and Pine Ridge. This on site help will relieve part of the burden on physicians at those service units and will hopefully help to retain those physicians by preventing burnout.

In addition, assuring a reliable referral service at Regional Hospital with familiar tribally hired physicians, who know the rural physicians and patients from their own outreach clinics, will reduce stress on the rural physicians, who will know whom to call in an emergency. The reverse is also true: the tribal ob-gyn physician, from having worked on site at the rural service unit, will know whom to call at that service unit to assure follow up of patients upon discharge from Regional Hospital.[37]

Thus, the RCIHB ob–gyn program is a potential model for Indian self-determination health care systems throughout the nation. Time will tell how the role of federal programs such as IHS may need to adapt to changing social and political forces, such as the 1994 Health Care Reform under

President Clinton. Responding to the demands of tribal and socioeconomic groups for health care equality requires caring physicians to take the lead in politics, economics, and public education in addition to simply treating disease.

SUMMARY

As our nation approaches a new era in health care, there are many lessons to be learned from the successes and failures of the past and from older cultures and traditional healers. If we are to work toward a better world, we must learn to respect the customs and beliefs of others. We must put on other people's shoes and view the world from their perspective. At the same time, we need to apply science toward conquering ill health, but we can do this only by adapting our methods so they are acceptable within other traditions and social contexts. The Navajos say that ill health occurs when man breaks harmony with Mother Earth, and good health cannot be restored until man is brought back into harmony and learns to walk in beauty. Perhaps, above all, we must learn to respect and protect Mother Earth and all her creatures and resources. Walk in beauty!

A TRIBUTE

This chapter is dedicated to the memory of three IHS physicians who were fighting for social change and lost their lives in the line of duty in a small plane crash while providing medical consultation to Indian patients and communities.

Dr. Ruggles Stahn, Diabetes Control Officer.
Dr. Chris Krogh, Maternal Child Health Consultant.
Dr. Arvo Oopik, Cardiologist.

Edie and Tom recruited these three physicians to work for the Aberdeen Area Indian Health Service and are struggling to carry on the work that they began.

POSTSCRIPT

Dr. Tom Welty continues to work as the Medical Epidemiologist for the Aberdeen Area Indian Health Service, serving over 100,000 Indian people in North Dakota, South Dakota, Iowa, and Nebraska. He serves as the Principal Investigator for several research projects including a study of cardiovascular disease among American Indians, a hepatitis A vaccine trial in infants and children, an infant mortality study to investigate the high rate of SIDS, and a study of breast and cervical cancer screening among Northern Plains Indians.

Dr. Edie Welty currently works as a Family Physician with the All Nations Clinic, a clinical program of the Rapid City Indian Health Board. She provides prenatal, obstetric, gynecologic, and newborn care to Indian patients from western South Dakota and travels several days a month to provide clinical services at Eagle Butte, South Dakota, located 180 miles from Rapid City.

Both physicians remain active in outdoor activities including trail running, mountain biking, and exploring remote areas of the western United States. Their older daughter Julie graduated from University of Minnesota Medical School in June 1995 and is providing voluntary service for public health programs in Latin America prior to starting a family practice residency in June 1997. Their younger daughter Anna, after graduation from Georgetown University, has worked at various jobs that allowed her to explore Alaska and Montana.

REFERENCES

1. Welty TK, Roberts EA: The effect of the attitude of examinee to examiner and the place of the exam in the casual blood pressures of Negro children aged 10–14, January 1967. Unpublished manuscript, University of Pittsburgh.
2. Dorris M: *The Broken Cord.* New York: Harper Perennial, 1990.
3. Duimstra C, Johnson D, Kutsch C, Wang B, Zentner M, Kellerman S, Welty TK: A fetal alcohol surveillance project in American Indian communities in the Northern Plains. *Public Health Rep* 1993;108:225–229.
4. Blendon RJ: Public health versus personal medical care; The dilemma of post-Mao China. *N Engl J Med* 1981;304:981–983.
5. Welty TK, Helgerson S, Tempest B, Gerber G, Johannes P: Control of tuberculosis among American Indians and Alaska Natives. *IHS Primary Care Provider* 1989;14:53–54.
6. Welty TK, Follas R: IHS standards of care for tuberculosis. INH preventive therapy. *IHS Primary Care Provider* 1989;14:54–58.
7. Mori MA, Leonardson G, Welty TK: The benefits of INH chemoprophylaxis and risk factors for tuberculosis among Oglala Sioux Indians. *Arch Intern Med* 1992;152:547–550.
8. Welty TK: Health survey of Sawmill, Arizona (a Navajo Indian community), summer 1967. Unpublished manuscript, University of Pittsburgh.
9. Van Duzen J, Carter JP, Zwagg RV: Protein and calorie malnutrition among preschool Indian children, a follow-up. *Am J Clin Nutr* 1976;29:657–662.
10. Coulehan JL, Lerner G, Helslsouer K, Welty TK, McLaughlin J: Acute myocardial infarction among Navajo Indians, 1976-83. *Am J Public Health* 1986;76:412–414.
11. Rhoades ER, Hammond J, Welty TK, Handler AO, Amler RW: The Indian burden of illness and future health interventions. *Public Health Rep* 1987;102:361–368.
12. Runkle B, Dahl R, Coulehan J, Michaels R, Welty TK, Cushing A: Summer diarrhea in an Indian population. *Ariz Med* 1983;40:228–230.
13. Tuttle J, Welty TK, Tauxe RV: Shigellosis: Treatment and prevention in Native American children. *IHS Primary Care Provider* 1992;117:117–121.
14. Welty TK, Hawk R, Rogers K: A program for correction of ear perforations in Navajo Indian children. *Public Health Rep* 1977;92:167–170.
15. Welty TK: *Special Needs of the Northern Plains American Indian Population. Report on Eye Research Planning Conference, Black Hills Regional Eye Institute, Rapid City, SD.* Oct. 21, 1989, pp. 16–22.

16. Welty TK, Grabman J, Kompare E, Welty E, Van Duzen J, Wood G, Rudd P, Poland J: Nineteen cases of plague in Arizona: A spectrum including ecthyma gangrenosum due to plague and plague in pregnancy. *West J Med* 1985;142:641–646.

17. Welty TK: Plague, method of Thomas Welty, M.D. In: Rakel RE, ed. *Conn's Current Therapy.* Philadelphia: WB Saunders, 1984:44–45.

18. Welty TK: Plague. *Am Fam Physician* 1986;33:159–164.

19. Stehr-Green P, Welty E, Burse V: Human exposure to polychlorinated biphenyls at toxic waste sites: Investigations in the United States. *Arch Environ Health* 1988;43:420–424.

20. Amler RW, Dull HB (eds.): *Closing the Gap — the Burden of Unnecessary Illness.* New York: Oxford University Press, 1987.

21. Welty TK, Freni LW, Zack MM, Weber P, Sippel J, Huete N, Justice J, Dever D, Murphy MA: Effects of exposure to salty drinking water in an Arizona community. Cardiovascular mortality, hypertension prevalence, and relationships between blood pressure and sodium intake. *JAMA* 1986;255:622–626.

22. Welty TK (ed.): *Indian Health Conditions.* Rockville, MD: Department of Health and Human Services, Public Health Service, Indian Health Service.

23. Oxen N, Bulterys M, Welty TK, Kraus JF: Sudden infant death among American Indians and whites in North and South Dakota. *Paediatr Perinat Epidemiol* 1990;4:177–185.

24. Welty TK: Cancer and cancer prevention and control programs in the Aberdeen Area Indian Health Service. *Am Indian Culture Res J* 1992;16:117–137.

25. Welty TK, Zephier N, Schweigman K, Blake B, Leonardson G: Cancer risk factors in three Sioux tribes: Use of the Indian-specific health risk appraisal for data collection and analysis. *Alaska Med* 1993,35:265–272.

26. Welty TK, Tanaka ES, Leonard B, Rhoades ER, Hurlburt WB, Fairbanks L: Indian Health Service facilities become smoke-free. *Morbid Mortal Week Rep* 1987;36:348–350.

27. Hrabovsky S, Welty TK, Coulehan J: Acute myocardial infarction and sudden death in Sioux Indians. *West J Med* 1989;150:420–422.

28. Welty TK, Lee ET, Yeh J, Cowen L, Fabsetz R, Le NA, Robbins D, Oopik A, Howard BV: Cardiovascular disease risk factors in American Indians. The Strong Heart Study. *Am J Epidemiol* 1995;142:269–287.

29. Welty TK: Health implictions of obesity in American Indians and Alaska Natives. *Am J Clin Nutr* 1991;53:1616S–1621S.

30. Welty TK, Coulehan JL: Cardiovascular disease among American Indians and Alaska Natives. *Diabetes Care* 1993;16(Suppl 1):277–283.

31. Welty TK: Indian-specific health risk appraisal developed. *IHS Primary Care Provider* 1988;13:65.

32. Welty TK: Finding the way — Indian-specific HRA released. *IHS Primary Care Provider* 1989;14:64–65.
33. Hammond J, Welty TK, Whirl Wind Soldier C, Condon R: Health promotion for Indian community leaders. *IHS Primary Care Provider* 1989;14:35–58.
34. Stanford Health Promotion Center and the Indian Health Service: *Restoring Balance — Community-Directed Health Promotion for American Indians and Alaska Natives.* Stanford: Stanford University Press, 1992.
35. Lee ET, Welty TK, Fabsitz R, Cowan LD, Le NA, Oopik AJ, Cucchiava AV, Savage PJ, Howard BV: The Strong Heart Study — A study of cardiovascular disease in American Indians: Design and methods. *Am J. Epidemiol* 1990;132:1141–1145.
36. Welty TK, Lee ET, Fabsitz R, Cowan LD, Le NA, Oopik AJ, Howard BV. The Strong Heart Study: A study of cardiovascular disease and its risk factors in American Indians. *IHS Primary Care Provider* 1992;17:32–33.
37. Welty ER: A potential solution for IHS problems in ob/gyn recruitment, retention and service delivery. *IHS Primary Care Provider* 1994;19:85–89.

CHAPTER IX

MY OBLIGATION
TO OTHERS

A Tradition Carried Forward

FERNANDO AURELIO SANCHEZ
MENDOZA, M.D., M.P.H.

I never considered myself an activist but rather an individual who was given the opportunity to help others. Having been given that opportunity, I felt obliged to take it; this tendency has guided my life to the present and in some ways shaped who and what I am today.

My sense of obligation to others came from my parents, Aurelio and Velia Mendoza. My father taught me through his words and actions, while my mother taught me through her emotions. Throughout my childhood my father explained to me that the reason to help others was *"para ser humano"* (to be human). This humanistic approach to life included a sense of right and wrong, but perhaps more importantly, it taught forgiveness and a willingness to care for others. For my father, seeing others suffer was a *"gran lastima"* (a great shame). My mother also expressed the importance of caring for others, but what I remember most was her empathy. When she saw others suffer, particularly children, she would become tearful and would do what she could to help. Through my parents I became aware of my responsibility to others, and this significantly colored my early world.

For my parents, family was the focus of existence. Success was measured not in material wealth but in the success and happiness of one's children. This cornerstone of Latino culture was embedded into both of my parents by my grandparents. Their intergenerational sense of family, tradition and obligation to others was our family's foundation. Therefore, to understand my choices in life, it is important to describe some of my family's background.

My grandfather fought in the Mexican Revolution and had been a Major in Pancho Villa's army. After the Revolution, he immigrated to the United States. He initially worked on the railroads in the Southwest but eventually settled in Fillmore, California, where he worked on a citrus farm. He had nine children; of these my father was the second oldest. My father was born in Mexico, came to the United States as an infant, and spent most of his childhood in Fillmore living in a farm workers camp. He attended a segregated school for the Mexican farm workers' children until the sixth grade. The white children attended a different school from the Mexican children; it was called *La Nueva Escuela* (the new school) because it was more esthetically pleasing. My father left school to support his family by working on the farm. At that time, the primary job opportunities for Mexican-Americans were in agriculture, as farm laborers. Frequently, even those who graduated from high school were unable to get better jobs, mostly because of discrimination against Mexican-Americans. For years afterward, my father would dream about going back to school and getting an education. Unfortunately for him, segregation and limited opportunities for Mexicans living in the United States were commonplace. His generation would not see the benefits of an education. This, I believe, forged his attitude toward education for his children.

My father's sense of commitment to others was nurtured by the example of his own father. In 1939, farm workers who worked on the citrus farms in southern California went on strike. The strike was organized by leaders of a national labor union and primarily involved the Mexican farm workers. My grandfather, who had worked 20 years for the same farmer, was asked not to go on strike by the owner of the farm. However, because my grandfather was one of the eldest members of his community, he decided to support his people and go on strike. At first, the union representatives were optimistic about winning the strike, but after a year their enthusiasm waned. The union withdrew its support of the farm workers, and the strike was defeated. My grandfather lost his job, his home, and his security. However, his family was intact. In 1942, he moved north to San Jose, California to work in the fruit orchards. Unfortunately, he died in 1947 before I was born, and I know him only through my father's stories.

I have mentioned my grandfather because he significantly influenced my father. Through stories about my grandfather, I was able to relate to the virtues of courage, responsibility, and leadership — virtues I also saw in my father. As a young boy growing up in the 1950s, and later as an adolescent in the 1960s, the idea of being related to someone who fought in the Mexican Revolution for the rights of the poor gave me a sense of continuity from the past to the present. This was reinforced when I was told that I looked like my grandfather.

During the time of the strike, my father sought jobs initially in Los Angeles and then in El Paso, Texas and Juarez, Mexico. It was there that he met my mother, the eldest in a family of four children. Although she had been born in El Paso, she spent her childhood and young adulthood in Juarez, Mexico, across the border from El Paso. Growing up in Juarez, she developed high self-esteem and a real awareness of her abilities — qualities her mother had fostered. My grandmother, a very determined, independent, and caring woman, was a role model for my mother. Her strength kept my mother's family together through difficult times. In the tradition of my grandmother, my mother transmitted the attributes of determination, independence, and caring for others to her children on a daily basis.

My mother loved to learn. Consequently, she always did well in school and graduated first in her high school class. After graduation, she put herself through night school in order to learn how to read and write English. This helped her obtain a job in El Paso to support her family. At this time, my mother was first exposed to the racism directed toward Mexicans living in the United States and to the conditions they lived in.

Shortly after my parents married, they returned to San Jose to rejoin my father's family. My father left agricultural work and became a truck driver, eventually buying his own truck. Ultimately, he ran his own trucking business, and by working 14-hour days became very successful. He then returned to farming as a second business, raising oranges and olives. In these business endeavors, my mother was his business manager and a key to his success. My parents achieved the American dream: they started with nothing, but through determination and hard work, they achieved success for themselves and their children. This was an example to all of us, and we took it to heart. Each of us fulfilled our parents' hopes by attending college. My brother Raymond is a lawyer, my brother Jaime is a social worker, and my sister Leticia is a college counselor. My brother Mario has his own trucking business, and my youngest brother, Aurelio Jr., is completing his college degree. This was the education that my father dreamed about and that my mother struggled to get for herself in her youth.

My mother encouraged learning and gave me support to succeed at anything that I tried. My father encouraged hard work, integrity, and loyalty to duty. Being an only child for seven years provided me with the opportunity to have my parents' attention focused on me during early childhood. Then, with the arrival of four brothers and one sister, I was given the responsibility to help raise my siblings. This responsibility, although trying at times, was the basis of my interest in children and pediatrics.

When I first started school, my parents and I lived in the basement of my paternal grandmother's house. It was located in a predominately low-income, Mexican-American neighborhood or *barrio* in the Gardner district of San Jose. My first language was Spanish, and my mother began to teach me English in preparation for kindergarten. My unfamiliarity with this new language made school challenging, but because most of the other children were in the same situation, I did not find myself an outsider. School was exciting and interesting. By the time I was in second grade, my father had saved enough money to buy his own house. We moved into a new neighborhood called Willow Glen, another suburb of San Jose that, unlike our former neighborhood, was a mixture of low-middle- to upper-income residential areas. We were one of only two Mexican-American families in the school district, so when I started at my new school, Booksin Elementary School, there was only one other Mexican-American child. I knew that I was different.

I made new friends quickly but found that because of my limited fluency in English, my school work suffered. I also began to stutter, which further limited my school performance. Reading out loud in class was highly stressful and an activity that I tried to avoid. I was required to repeat the third grade because of concern about my reading performance. Although this was difficult for me, my mother was very supportive and did not allow me to think that I was a failure. My other major setback occurred at the beginning of sixth grade. I had been elected class president and felt very proud that my classmates wanted me as their leader. The day after

the election, however, a combined class of fifth and sixth
graders was formed by the school. Those sixth graders, including me, who were less proficient in reading were placed
in this class. For me, this resulted in an added disappoint-
ment — removal as class president. It seemed very unfair at
the time, and I was left wondering whether I would ever succeed at anything. Fortunately, the class was taught by Mr.
Harold Threewit, a teacher who would change the way I
would think about myself for the rest of my life.

Mr. Threewit had been my teacher the previous year. I
had enjoyed his class, but returning seemed like a defeat.
Yet, the true teacher is one who can give perspective to the
world and can make a student feel competent in that world.
Mr. Threewit did this for me. He was sympathetic about my
loss but also made sure that I did not feel incompetent. I
have never forgotten the day when Mr. Threewit was quizzing
the class on arithmetic and I raised my hand to answer a
problem. He told me to put down my hand because I already
knew the answer. It was the first time that I was identified
as being academically outstanding. From that time on, my
strength in mathematics gave me self-confidence in school
and allowed me to pursue my eventual interest in science
and medicine.

A few years ago, I wrote to Mr. Threewit to thank him
for his support some 30 years ago. Our relationship, which
perhaps was of little significance to him, had had an immense
impact on my life. I had had a number of negative experiences during my elementary school years, but it took just one
positive experience to change my life. Mr. Threewit showed
me that a teacher can have a significant impact on a student
even though the effects may not be visible until many years
later. The good teacher has the faith to believe this is true;
I believe Mr. Threewit had this faith.

Junior high school was a time of personal transformation
and national transition. John F. Kennedy had just given his
famous inaugural speech about "what you can do for your

country." He had also resolved to place a man on the moon by the end of the decade. President Kennedy challenged us not only to accomplish earthly goals, such as ending poverty and hunger, but to achieve other goals that would take us into the future. To an adolescent, this emphasis on science as the road to the future was exciting.

However, the world of that day was also unpredictable. President Kennedy was assassinated. I saw police and their dogs chasing down men, women, and children during civil rights marches. I saw the plight of migrant farm workers living in dilapidated shacks. And I saw the beginning of a war in Vietnam. The world and society seemed to be in tremendous upheaval, and I saw it every evening on my television set. My generation was the most informed generation up to that time, and we were also the most challenged. The images on the screen were a powerful catalyst. But as a young adolescent, I had only a glimmering of understanding about what they meant.

I entered Willow Glen High School in 1965, the year after the Beatles made their national debut. San Francisco was becoming a Mecca for the new rock and roll music. High school students were being introduced to new music from home and abroad, and to new ways of thinking about society and life. The free speech movement was starting at Berkeley, and Joan Baez was beginning her career as an activist and folk singer. Cesar Chavez began organizing activities in San Jose. The calm and order of the 1950s had turned into a time of questioning and doubt. Adolescence is always a time to find one's identity, but the events of that time heightened my sense of adventure.

Friendships are important to adolescents, and they were for me. My friendship with Tom Farris, which began during that time, has lasted for 32 years. I first met Tom in seventh grade during Spanish class. Tom came from a middle-class family, but despite our different cultures we shared similar values. His parents would always welcome me to his home, and my parents would do the same. He loved Mexican food — and in particular my mother's cooking. His mother always found something to smile about and was one of the most pleasant people I have ever met. His father was a graduate of Stanford University, but what I remember most was his expertise at barbecuing. I suppose if I ever had a second family, they were it. From my friendship with Tom, I learned that one can have a relationship with someone from another cultural background based on commonalties rather than differences. This is a lesson that I have tried to use in all my interactions with others: looking for commonalties in order to develop a personal link with other individuals.

However, I have learned that sometimes this strategy does not work because for some, differences are more important. This was reinforced when one day a friend of several years, while bantering with a group of his friends, asked me what type of blood I had. When I responded B positive, he and his friends laughed. It was only later that I realized that he was inquiring about whether I was a Mexican. Although Willow Glen High School was generally a heterogeneous environment, as in most high schools, cliques and group affiliations were important. Most of the Mexican-American students came from lower socioeconomic backgrounds, and this distinction separated them from many of the other students. This contributed to a perception that being Mexican-American was second class. Although I came from a lower socioeconomic background, I did not consider myself second class. I knew that I could compete well in science and mathematics, and I had a strong positive sense of my culture. Therefore, I decided to show that Mexicans were as capable as anyone else. Looking back now, it was in Mr. Threewit's class that I discovered that I could do well academically, but in high school I began to develop a purpose for that success — to show that a Mexican-American could achieve. Although I was not the top student in the school, I was academically successful enough to impress my fellow students and teachers. To show that I could do something when others said it was impossible has been a strong motivating force in my life.

The Mexican-American population in San Jose was about 20%, and my high school had about 5% to 10% Mexican-American students. Other high schools in San Jose, however, had much larger populations of Mexican-American students (from 20% to 50%). Juxtaposed to the high proportion of Mexican-American students in local high schools were very low percentages of Mexican-American students in local colleges, usually less than 2%. Therefore, although voting rights for Mexican-Americans in California were not the issue they were for African-Americans in other parts of the country, educational and economic opportunity were. It seemed that the only way to improve this situation would be to increase the number of Mexican-American students entering college. To accomplish this goal, various organizations encouraged Mexican-American high school students to attend college. One of those groups, the Mexican-American Youth Organization (MAYO), was brought to our high school by college students from San Jose State College.

MAYO started with Elena Hernandez as president and me serving as vice-president. Elena was a Mexican-American student who had come from a background similar to mine. She was tough, determined, smart, and a natural leader. Although I felt at ease in the classroom, it was stressful for me to be in a position of leadership, particularly when it required public speaking. My stuttering had been somewhat controlled with speech therapy, but it was evident in any stressful situation. Therefore, I tried to avoid any public speaking unless I felt that the issues were important enough to overcome my shortcomings. Elena and I organized a group of approximately ten Mexican-American students, and developed city-wide events to encourage students to go to college. Elena was very passionate about improving the status of the Mexican-American community. She truly felt the injustice and prejudice that Mexican-Americans lived with each day.

For her, MAYO was not just some high school club, it was a social movement. If the difference between a Mexican-American and a Chicano is actively contributing to the sociopolitical movement, then she was the first Chicana I encountered. Her passion rubbed off on me, and the following year I was the president of MAYO. At that point my desire for social change had overcome my self-doubts about leadership.

Another event that changed my life happened when I was in the 11th grade. One day, my counselor called me into her office and said that she had heard I wanted to be a doctor. This was the first time I had ever thought about being a doctor! In fact, up to that point, I had planned to be a chemist. My counselor asked me if I would like to attend a conference for high school students interested in careers in health. The idea of being a doctor intrigued me, and I went. There, the details of how one becomes a doctor were explained, and for the first time, a career as a physician became a possibility for me. I had had some contact with physicians, because two of my friends' fathers had been physicians. However, medicine as a career had not yet entered my mind. Perhaps it was at that point that my interest in science intersected with my interest in helping people; medicine seemed like the most rational choice. It also seemed that pediatrics would be an appropriate choice because I had had considerable experience with children. But perhaps the real reason that pediatrics seemed enticing was that it worked with the future . . . children.

I graduated from Willow Glen High School in June 1967 and the following fall entered San Jose State College as a biochemistry major. College was relatively uneventful for me. San Jose State College was primarily a commuter school, and I lived at home in order to save money for medical school. During the summer and school vacations, I worked at a variety of different jobs. I was a janitor, foundry worker, and truck driver; however, during the school year I did not work. My father was willing to support me in order to insure that I did well. I did not want to let him down, so I studied hard.

During the 4 years at San Jose State, the world changed. The Vietnam War was in full swing. Many of my high school friends were either being drafted or were joining the armed services. Those of us in college initially received deferments, but as the war began to escalate, we were placed in a lottery. War protest marches were commonplace on campus during that time. Like many others, I was concerned about the war. Although I had been brought up to respect our country and defend it, I was having trouble understanding why we were fighting in Vietnam. If I had been drafted, it would have been difficult to decide what to do. Could I ever justify killing another human being? The decision was made for me; my lottery number was 256 — putting me out of the draft range.

However, the war did affect me through the death of a family member. Rudy Renterria was the brother of my aunt and had been an all-city basketball star. He was someone whom everyone liked, the all-American kid. Rudy had been given a basketball scholarship to a local college but decided not to attend. As a result, he was drafted into the Army. His tour of duty was just about up when he was killed. At his funeral, there was deep sadness that someone so full of life and with such a bright future had to die so young. It could have happened to me if I had not been in college. I wondered about my responsibility to the country as one who had not gone to war.

At that time, the other great events on campus revolved around the civil rights movement. In 1968, San Jose State, like most colleges in the nation, had marches and student rallies to support the civil rights movement. At first, the protests were nonviolent. But after the assassination of Martin Luther King, speakers began to promote more aggressive action. Certainly, it was the easiest way to handle the anger that many felt about society's inability to correct injustices. It was clear that these problems had developed over many years and were not going to be resolved with any "quick fix" approach, either peaceful or violent. I recalled the history of my family and the racial prejudice they had had to overcome. I recalled the "American" ideals that I grew up with in the 1950s — the sense that America was fair and that sacrifice and hard work would be rewarded. Yet, I knew that for the families of those Chicanos who fought in Vietnam, whether or not the soldiers came back or died there, participation in the American dream was not a certainty. I asked myself "would the next generation of Chicanos have it better than the generation that fought in this war?" As I looked around, the answer seemed to be no. Not without significant changes for Chicanos.

I decided that I would try to improve the lives of Chicano children. I had no grandiose plan to change the world, but I thought that if I could become a pediatrician, I could at least help improve Chicano children's health. I refocused my efforts to get into medical school and began to inform myself about the health concerns of the Chicano community.

While in college, I became friends with Hector Ramón, a Chicano student who came from a similar lower-middle-class background. Hector and I shared the experience of being evaluated by others: were we "Chicano," that is, politically correct? This assessment was particularly common during the late 1960s and early 1970s, when "if you weren't part of the solution, you were part of the problem." For many, being an activist meant going into the streets and protesting. Hector saw the world differently, yet had as much passion for helping Chicanos as anyone I knew. He saw change as changing the world outside the campus, in the community. For him, change and improvement would come when Chicanos were lawyers, doctors, and individuals who owned their own businesses. Although very much a pragmatist, he had a heart for others. He reinforced my thinking about what I wanted to do with my life and also helped to clarify for me that real change must involve the community and not just words on a college campus. Hector went on to Harvard Law School and subsequently returned to San Jose to practice law in the Latino community. I went to Stanford Medical School and began my new life.

My first contact with medical school began during the summer after my graduation from San Jose State College. Chris Murlas, a second-year Stanford medical student, invited me to join a group of Stanford medical students who were interested in working with the Gardner Community Center in San Jose. This organization wanted to start a neighborhood health center and sought help from the county medical society. Through the president of the medical society, Dr. Skilcorn, Chris had become involved with the Center's efforts. Along with three other students, Chris had the support of Dr. William Fowkes, a Stanford faculty member and Director of the Regional Medical Program (RMP).

This was an opportunity that seemed too good to be true. I was not only going to be working in the neighborhood where I spent my childhood, but I would be providing an important link between the Chicano community and the Stanford medical community. I was the only Chicano medical student, which thrust me into the unique position of interpreter and mediator. Although my knowledge of medicine at this point was nonexistent, my knowledge about the community and its people proved very useful. My job was to listen to the people of the Gardner community, taking care not to supersede their concerns and interests with what I thought was important.

I was helped in this task by the head of the Gardner Community Center, Jim Flores. Jim was an ex-paratrooper who had self-confidence about his abilities to lead but made a significant effort to listen to the concerns of all community members. He, along with Mr. Hugo Jimenez, another senior local resident active in the Gardner community, was my mentor. At times there were disagreements between the Gardener and Stanford groups. However, I learned that process and not outcome was the most important part of developing a neighborhood health center. The only way this type of health center could exist and function was if the community felt empowered and saw the health center as their own. Otherwise, the health center would be just like any other clinic established by an outside institution: something that was there physically but not really part of the community's spirit.

For us, empowerment meant that those most affected by the clinic should decide its goals, function, and governance. Even for our group of liberal-minded medical students and faculty, this was sometimes hard to do. Although the health center belonged to the community, we felt we had a claim to it because of the significant physical and emotional effort our student group had invested. This became a particularly sticky problem when community politics started to play a part in the decision-making process, leading to factions in the community group. In the final analysis, the community health center would survive only if it had the support of all its community members. Factions would have to agree that the most important thing was to keep the health center functioning. This lesson in compromise was important for all of us. For me, it began my instruction on how to be an intermediary between the community and an institution.

I continued to work with the clinic during my first year in medical school, and then into the following summer. By that time, the Center's community board had hired a well-respected community organizer, Mr. Michael Kilpatrick. The health center's facility was initially a closed Catholic school located on the grounds of the Scared Heart Church. Later, the monsignor of the church, Father Healy, allowed us to move the health center to an old rectory building. After helping remodel the rectory with the other students, I was given the opportunity through RMP to do a survey of ten community health clinics in California. I wanted to see if the Gardner Health Center's experience was similar to those of other neighborhood health centers. It was exciting to travel to urban and rural clinics and to meet others interested in community health. But it was also enlightening. Perhaps for the first time, I realized that alternative health care risked becoming second-class health care. Among the health centers I visited, I saw some that totally depended on volunteer medical personnel and donated drugs and equipment. Many had great difficulty hospitalizing their patients because no one would take them. In contrast, others had managed to become part of the regular health care system, though sometimes only peripherally. The latter seemed to be financially stable and to meet the needs of their communities with good quality health care. This observation convinced me that community health centers need to connect themselves with the "regular" health care system in order to be successful. Over the next few years, with combined efforts from the community board, Mike Kilpatrick, and the Stanford medical students and faculty, the Gardner Health Center established links with its local health care system. Twenty years later, the Gardner Health Center is still serving its community and providing high-quality care.

The other significant experience for me during this time had to do with the Catholic church. Although I had been raised a Catholic and believed myself to be religious, my experience with religion had been mixed. Once my mother had gone to the monsignor of our parish to ask for help for a group of migrant farm workers but was refused because they did not belong to the parish. To me, this seemed contradictory to the church's teachings. I came to believe that organized religion was more concerned with its institutional structure than with its teachings. Fortunately, the work at the Gardner Health Center introduced me to a group of priests who were living their religion. The monsignor, Father Healy, and the parish priests committed their lives to improving the physical and spiritual lives of their community. Father Healy and his priests were involved with Cesar Chavez's protest marches to fight for farm worker's rights. They worked with community activists to improve the living conditions within the low-income Gardner community. Father Healy even closed the church's Catholic school and turned it into a neighborhood education center for local children and adults; while the Catholic school had been successful, it had been serving the needs of middle- and upper-class families outside the community. Father Healy believed that a church needed to serve its community and the poor first, so he directed his church's resources toward these groups.

These priorities rekindled my interest in the Catholic church. I realized that any institution is only as effective as the people involved in it and that one person can make a significant difference given the position to create change and the determination to accomplish it. Father Healy and his assistant, Father Isaac, both showed me that this was possible. Yet their greatest lesson was that religion was something that should be lived rather than just discussed or held within.

Medical school was hard but exciting. Again there seemed to be the need to prove myself to my classmates. The two medical school classes prior to my own had been the first with minority students admitted through affirmative action. In my class, we had ten minority students: five African-Americans, four Mexican-Americans, and one Native American. Although most students and faculty treated us well, there were some who expressed concern about our capabilities. Thus, we all felt that we needed to work hard to prove ourselves. My Chicano classmates Alex Rodarte, Jose Santos, and Antonio Ruiz, and I worked together to insure our success. In so doing, we helped each other mature and develop as medical students and became life-long friends. One of the main reasons for our success was our belief in each other: we knew that we were not second-class students. Our conviction that minority students should have the opportunity to become physicians made us committed to the expansion of the affirmative action program at Stanford Medical School. Jose, Alex, Antonio, and I all became involved with the recruitment and admission of minority medical students. This was my first experience with the inner workings of medical education. I came to understand the gatekeeping process of medical schools and the importance of being part of that process in order to increase the number of minority physicians.

Overall, my medical school years were enjoyable. During the second and third years, I shared a house with three other classmates: Fred Heindrick, Dan Walker, and John Koabashi. Each of us was quite different from the others. Fred was a kind and gentle person who had broad interests. He not only took classes to improve his Spanish but also gained fluency in Chinese. Dan, from Great Falls, Montana, was an excellent country folk singer who brought out his guitar and started singing cowboy songs whenever he was down. John was from Texas, where his father was a truck farmer. He was a serious student but was always willing to help others with a problem. This group helped me appreciate other points of view; we had many discussions about thorny issues that would have not been possible if we had not been good friends and roommates.

The clinical years initially were difficult. They forced me to be comfortable with speaking in public, even when I stuttered. Moreover, fitting into the clinical team was sometimes taxing. For example, during my medical rotation, I was asked by my senior resident what my father did. When I responded that he was a truck driver, the resident expressed surprise because he had not met a student with that kind of background. Although I got along well with other team members, I always felt like a social outsider. Yet I knew that if I were to succeed in medicine, I would need to fit into the system.

During my pediatric rotation, my oral presentations were not going well, partially because of my speech impediment. The clerkship director called me into her office and told me that I should think about another field. I felt saddened but told her that pediatrics was my chosen field and that I would work hard to improve my presentations. Although I got some support from my friends, I mostly worked on my own to improve my clinical presentations. I forced myself to overcome my concerns about how I sounded and concentrated on what

I wanted to say. This was a personal battle that only I could win or lose, but one that was eased by having the support of friends and faculty members. Although my stuttering has never completely gone away, it is one nemesis that I have been able to control. A personal success!

Alex, Jose, and I graduated in 1975 from Stanford Medical School and entered the pediatric residency program at Stanford Hospital together. We all did well and went on to productive careers. Today, Alex is a pediatric anesthesiologist at the Children's Hospital in San Diego and president of the largest anesthesia group in the country. Jose is a professor of pediatrics and Director of the Department of Infectious Diseases at the Children's Hospital in Mexico City. Antonio is successfully practicing internal medicine in San Antonio, Texas. Each has contributed significantly to improving the health of people. Looking back, I had no doubt that they would be successful doctors. If they had not been given the chance to succeed, our world would be the lesser for it now.

Pediatric residency was very enjoyable. While the work was hard, there was something very satisfying about helping children and their families. At the same time, it became clear to me that medical technology could do only so much to improve the health of children. I became aware that the socioeconomic status of children's families and their parents' abilities to parent were sometimes as important as prescribed medications in improving children's health. If I truly was going to improve the health care of children, particularly those who were poor and Latino, then I had to broaden my perspective of health care. For this reason, after my residency, I decided to obtain a Masters in Public Health. I wanted to understand better the sociocultural issues related to children's health and to prepare myself to deal with the health care issues of Latino children.

The other major event in my life during residency was that I met and married my wife, Alicia. I first saw her at a party for Latino medical students. I called her for a blind date, and luckily, she accepted. Alicia was from Mexico City and had lived there until she was 20, when she moved to California. Her father was Mexican and her mother American. She had grown up in a Mexican culture but felt very comfortable in the American culture. Although we had a common cultural background that helped us understand each other, our differences made our marriage interesting. She was interested in art and animals, particularly horses. I, in turn, had my interest in medicine and the Chicano movement. In any marriage, it is important to have things one can share and things that are unique that add to the other person's life. Our marriage has been an exploration of these two areas. We were married at the Sacred Heart Church in San Jose by Father Healy. It seemed an appropriate place to start a new life.

A few months after we got married, we traveled to Boston, where I enrolled in the public health school at Harvard University. I took classes in maternal and child health to learn the public health approach to dealing with children's health problems. I found that very little was known about minority children's health status, particularly for Latino children. I was, however, fortunate to meet Dr. Robert Haggerty who was one of the first academic General Pediatricians in the country. I explained my interest, and the dilemma of not being able to find information about the health status of Latino children. I also informed him that I was somewhat torn between going into public health to be an administrator versus remaining in clinical medicine. He suggested an alternative, a career in academic medicine. Dr. Haggerty explained to me that I could do research on the health issues of Latino children, and at the same time, continue to be involved in clinical medicine by teaching students and residents. I had not thought about this alternative, but it seemed a reasonable solution to my problem. Fortunately, Dr. Haggerty had just become the Director of the Robert Wood Johnson General Pediatric Academic Development Fellowship. This fellowship was intended to train General Pediatricians in research to allow them to pursue an academic career. One of the fellowship programs was at Stanford University in the Department of Pediatrics. I contacted the Chairman of the Department and the Program Director, and was accepted into the program. Alicia and I returned home.

Although I learned some research methodology while at the public health school, the fellowship provided me with the foundation for my future clinical research endeavors. My fellowship research project examined the social support systems of families with asthmatic children. The project successfully showed that asthmatic children with good social support systems used emergency room services less. After the fellowship, I was asked to assume a faculty position in the Department of Pediatrics. At first, I wasn't sure whether this position would enable me to work on behalf of Latino children. Somehow, it seemed a long way away from my interest in community medicine. Nevertheless, in July 1981, I joined the Stanford Medical School faculty and was the only minority faculty member at the Medical School.

When I first became a faculty member, it was as if I was an adolescent again, since I felt I had to learn the "right" things to do in this "faculty society." Moreover, as before, I was a minority in a new area, and I did not want to fail. I worked hard, thinking that this would overcome any shortcomings. I now focused my research more directly on Latino children. I first collaborated in a research project with another colleague in which we examined the verbal interaction between prenatal care providers and pregnant adolescents who were Latinas: Mexican and Mexican-Americans. We housed the project at the Stanford Center for Chicano Research, a recently formed research center focusing on the Chicano community. This began my long-term association with the Chicano Research Center.

My next project involved an assessment of the Hispanic Health and Nutrition Examination Survey (HHANES). This health survey specifically targeted Mexican-Americans, mainland Puerto Ricans, and Cuban-Americans, and was conducted by the National Center for Health Statistics. This provided me with the research opportunity that I had been seeking: a chance to increase information about Latino children that could have an immediate effect on health policies. The HHANES project also allowed me to work with Reynaldo Martorell, a professor at the Food Research Institute at Stanford. Rey was an outstanding scholar who had an international reputation in assessing the growth and development of children. He was from Honduras and, as a Latino, had a strong interest in the Latino population in the United States. Therefore, although his previous work had been in Latin America, he was very enthusiastic about working with me on the HHANES project. Over the years, Rey has been a mentor, a colleague, and a close friend. As a young faculty member, I was still "learning the ropes of the trade," and Rey was there to assist me. He helped me get through the adolescence phase of my academic career and to develop a sense of what it is to be a faculty member. For this, I will alway be thankful.

Our HHANES research group included investigators from other universities, and not only produced a variety of publications on Latino children's health and nutritional status but also communicated findings to the general public and to policy makers. Information from HHANES conferences and from our articles was published in the *Washington Post* and other newspapers, and local television sought out our group for our opinions. I testified to Congress on the nutritional needs of Latino children. My conjecture that the media increasingly wanted information on Latino children was confirmed.

In September 1990, I became the Director of the Stanford Center for Chicano Research. Although my research projects had been housed at this institute since 1983, I had not been involved with its administration. The Center's previous

research agenda included cultural studies, literature, and
policy studies; as the new Director, I reexamined this
agenda. The Latino population throughout the country was
increasing dramatically. Therefore, I reasoned that any study
having to do with our present society would, *de facto,* be a
study of Chicanos/Latinos if they were a significant percent-
age of the study's population. For example, a study of California, where approximately 25% of the population is Latino,
would also be a study of Latinos. Conveying this perspective
to other faculty significantly expanded the Center's fields of
research. One project explored how pesticides and lead in
the environment may significantly affect the health and development of children of farm workers. Another examined
the style of management in large successful companies and
the treatment of Latinos in the work force. Still another analyzed how the media depicts Latino culture and makes suggestions about how to reduce bias.

These approaches to research in the Chicano community
were mutlidisciplinary and focused on critical problems for
all of society. These studies expanded the relevance of Chi-
cano/Latino research to all Americans by examining issues
that affect many groups in society. I hoped our newfound
knowledge would empower the Chicano/Latino community. I
also hoped that our work would encourage students to see
research as exciting and with potential to affect the real
world.

Throughout my career, I have tried to recruit and develop
minority medical students. In 1983, I was appointed Assistant
Dean of Student Affairs in the School of Medicine. Because
I was the only minority on the medical school faculty, I believed that I needed to support the minority medical students.
In retrospect, it was probably not the best decision because
of the large time commitment. Yet, we all make choices based
not just on our intellect but also on our emotions. For me,
service to others was a greater call than academic accomplishment. I was the only minority faculty at the medical

school, and this, I felt, bestowed on me a responsibility to help those coming behind me. Over the years, I have questioned this decision but have never regretted it. I recall the example of Mr. Threewit, who was there at a critical time in my life and helped me without knowing it. I hope that I have been able to do the same for some of my students.

As in my academic career, I have been privileged to have colleagues who served as mentors. Doctors Roy Maffly, John Steward, and Robert Cutler were all Associate Deans who supported and encouraged my career in medical education. With their help, I tried to meet the needs of minority medical students at Stanford Medical School.

At first, I focused on recruiting minority students to the school and on providing academic and personal counseling to them once they arrived. Although their matriculation and graduation rates were both high, I realized that most minority medical students were missing an important opportunity to participate in the research opportunities available at Stanford Medical School. As a result, they were developing fewer mentor relationships with faculty and were less likely to have an interest in academic medicine. I initially thought that minority medical students should return to their communities to practice, but I came to feel that minority physicians were needed in all areas of medicine, especially in academic medicine. This was particularly true for Chicanos, because in 1983 there were only 63 Mexican-American medical school faculty members out of the 50,000 medical school faculty in the United States.

My research activities had demonstrated that health information on Chicanos and Latinos was almost nonexistent, and without more Latino faculty to do research, this was unlikely to change. Therefore, under the guidance of Dr. Robert Cutler, and with the help of my colleagues, Drs. Patricia Cross, Ronald Garcia, and Carl Rhodes, we instituted the Early Matriculation Program for minority medical students. This program dramatically increased the numbers of minority medical students who did research and those who pursued academic careers. The program also did something that I had not anticipated: it increased the self-confidence of minority students. Although they still felt that they were different, they nonetheless believed that they were part of the institution.

The message about the importance of minority faculty, and the need to increase the number of minorities in all fields of medicine, was one that I discussed with my minority counterparts at other medical schools and with staff at the Association of American Medical Colleges. Unfortunately, this message was sometimes superseded by the need to recruit more minority physicians into primary care. Over the years I have become more resolute in my conviction that all fields of medicine must be integrated before the health care system will be truly responsive to minority needs.

Recently, I was promoted to Associate Dean and was awarded a Centers of Excellence grant from the federal government to help support minority student recruitment and retention, minority health care research facilitation, and minority faculty development. This has opened new avenues for me and my colleagues in the areas of medical education. In the new environment of health care reform, this grant will help me promote change in the medical school environment. Under these circumstances, I believe that new opportunities will exist to make the medical school environment more diverse and sensitive to the needs of all people. Stanford Medical School provides not only a supportive environment for this change to take place but also high visibility in medical education. I hope that I will be able to meet this challenge.

Finally, throughout my career, I have had a very supportive wife, a close family, and caring friends. This has allowed me to pursue my various interests. Without them, I would not have succeeded. Still there has been a cost. My wife and I have three lovely children, Julia, Fernando, and Carla. Julia is currently 13 years old and enjoys every bit of life. Fernando is 11 years old and is referred to as my clone because he looks like me and is quiet, caring, and eager to please. Carla is 8 years old and is a very determined little girl but is also quite sensitive. Looking back on my career, I realize that I have not participated in their lives as much as I would have wanted. As a result of travel, deadlines, and a sense of obligation to the job and minority issues, I have sacrificed family time. Unfortunately, when one is focused on short-term goals and deadlines, long-term goals — such as being part of a family — can be compromised. This sometimes happens without much awareness, particularly when the sense of mission becomes too strong.

This past year I was on sabbatical, and I had a chance to reflect on my career and my life. I thought about what I would be doing over the next 10 to 20 years. Although I believe that my career has had social relevance and has been very satisfying, personal satisfaction has not necessarily come from those activities. Instead, feeling that I have "missed opportunities" to participate in my family's life has made me reevaluate my career and commitments. I have come to believe that in order to have complete satisfaction, personal satisfaction must also be prioritized. I am sure that I will continue to meet my obligation to improve the health of the Latino community. However, I now see this obligation as a longer-term commitment that must be better integrated into the rest of my life.

If I were going to give advice to those interested in becoming social activists, I would say to them that there are many opportunities in the world today. Need is ubiquitous. One should select one issue that is personally relevant, so that a true long-term commitment can be made. If no issue is forthcoming, then one's personal experiences with those in need should be expanded. Professional commitment can be sustained over time only if personal satisfaction and happiness are present. I have learned that a balance between both important aspects of life — career and family — must be actively maintained. I believe achieving this balance will yield the greatest benefits for myself and the family members, friends, and community that comprise my world.

POSTSCRIPT

Dr. Fernando Mendoza still serves on the faculty of the Stanford University School of Medicine Department of Pediatrics. Over the past year, changes in California legislation have heightened his concern about the welfare of minority children and their families. Although disheartened by our political climate, he continues working to improve children's lives through clinical, research, and policy work. As Associate Dean of Student Affairs, Dr. Mendoza seeks to maintain the best of affirmative action in a national environment increasingly hostile to this policy. Dr. Mendoza reports that his family has been and remains a source of pleasure and sustenance.

CHAPTER X

TRYING TO MAKE A DIFFERENCE

JOHN E. MACK, M.D.

Those who dream by night in the dusty recesses of their minds wake in the day to find that all was vanity; but the dreamers of the day are dangerous men, for they may act their dream with open eyes, and make it possible.

— T. E. Lawrence, *Seven Pillars of Wisdom,* 1935

An invitation to write of the facts of one's life and the forces that have driven and shaped them presents for me, at 64, a special challenge and opportunity. Any attempt to provide coherence to events and experiences that seemed, while they were being lived, not only to lack unity and clear direction but to feel at times quite random or chaotic must to a degree represent a false imposition of order. Yet, I suppose, all learning and teaching must to some extent be like that. For if we are to pass our experience — and, yes, lessons — on to others we must make them tangible and give them form, creating, if we can, a story from which meaning might be derived.

This is a book about physicians who have fought for social change. I am pleased to be identified that way and can see that such struggles have been an important part of my life. But at the same time, the assignment has piqued a certain curiosity, a self-questioning. It has made me wonder about the roots of these efforts and inspired a desire to look inward and explore the soil from which they have grown.

In order for social actions to be effective, they must, I think, grow out of some context or tradition that enables others to recognize their own desires and potentialities, some undercurrent of larger purpose with which they may connect. Otherwise actions that are directed toward social or political change may appear as isolated behaviors, outside of our appropriate role or competence. In the course of their education and specialty training, physicians are consciously and unconsciously drawn into an ethos of healing, a commitment to trying to reduce suffering, and a dedication to human betterment. But the expression of these purposes may occur at the individual or the collective level, as in the field of public health.

Participants in the physicians' antinuclear movement, for example, represented by groups such as Physicians for Social Responsibility and International Physicians for the Prevention of Nuclear War, were always quick to connect their efforts to public service and public health traditions and described the nuclear arms race in the language of those disciplines. This would be, we said, "the last epidemic,"[1] and one of the most effective arguments that we could present to the public concerned the fact that only prevention was possible. Treatment after a nuclear war was utterly beyond our capability, we showed, at symposia that were attended by hundreds of thousands of anxious citizens. Although this approach was seen by conservatives who were unhappy with the political implications of the message to be stretching the limits of the medical mandate, it was important to maintain a link to our professional base. When we were seen as too nakedly political, our efforts were easier to discredit.

But this outlining of professional traditions, and the derivation of actions from them, does not say much about what makes a particular person at specific moments in history engage in certain issues of the time. For this we need to know about that person, his or her cultural background, formative influences, and private motivations, what is called, in the shorthand of our time, his identity. But a word of caution is needed here, a reminder of the incompleteness of retrospection and reflection. A mystery will remain, and explanations are inadequate. We can wonder and examine, but, finally, there is much that we do that seems beyond our ability to understand.

The expansion of the scope of social commitment has paralleled the evolution of my own psychospiritual development. As I have come increasingly to see myself as connected beyond human relationships and have grown to feel a kind of oneness within the expanse of creation, I have become increasingly interested in the dangers of ecological devastation and, finally, in the problems of consciousness that have restricted human ability to experience life and meaning beyond the boundaries of the earth. I have come to see the major social problems of our time — economic inequality, environmental destruction, and ethnonational conflicts that might escalate to a nuclear holocaust — as deriving from a too narrow definition of ourselves, a kind of psychospiritual bankruptcy that permits, and even encourages, exploitation at every level of existence. But more of that later.

I wonder if any subculture has developed the use of the intellect — some say at the expense of other faculties — further than the German Jewish people from whom I am descended. Freud, Marx and Einstein were German Jews, and there was never any doubt that my English professor father and economist mother expected me to become some sort of an academic. But there are other traditions among the German Jews of collective responsibility and community service, well exemplified by my father's family, who settled in Cincinnati, Ohio in the mid-19th century. Over several generations these forebears devoted themselves to a remarkable variety of charitable and cultural activities in the fields of child care, art, music, and religion, including the founding of a temple, hospital, and orphanage. My great-grandfather was an ophthalmologist who pioneered the use of anesthetics in eye surgery, and a great uncle, Joseph Aub, was one of the first Jewish professors of medicine at Harvard Medical School.

The image of medicine was actually *too* activist for me when I was growing up, not as intellectual a profession (there would certainly be *some* profession) as I expected to enter. Furthermore, my mother, in her authoritative way, seemed to boss our pediatrician — the only doctor I really knew — around like the tradesmen who came to the house to fix the plumbing or the stove. Yet there was also a part of me that protested secretly against the heady, wordy discussions of books and plays at the dinner table. The social issues of our times were endlessly talked about, especially the events in Europe that culminated in World War II and the Holocaust, leaving me with a terrible feeling of helplessness. For no one ever seemed to *do* anything about the problems that were so richly and excitedly discussed. This was, of course, unfair, for both of my parents were involved in various charities, and teaching and research were certainly respectable ways of contributing to human well-being. At the same time, too, my parents, while avoiding with disdain (I now suspect out of anxiety) what they called "administration," were passing on values of social commitment so that I might some day be able to live a few of their unlived lives.

Then there was my mother's brother, Julius ("Bud") Prince, whose attendance in medical school when I was a small boy seemed to carry a certain worthy mystique. Uncle Bud later became a famous public health doctor who battled for the development of health care systems in Ghana and Ethiopia. He is the most indefatigable activist doctor I know and surely, though I did not know it growing up, became some sort of role model. When I was 20, my sister, Mary Lee (also an academic, with a Ph.D. in economics and a masters in public health), married Sidney Ingbar, who became perhaps the world's leading thyroidologist and one of Harvard's most eminent professors of medicine. Sid became like a brother to me — I had no other — and though he was not a social activist my nearly daily contact with him before and especially during medical school (at Harvard, where Joe Aub helped me get in) allowed me to appreciate ever more profoundly the range of possibilities that medicine offered.

Throughout my adolescence and continuing up to the present time, my uncle Saul Scheidlinger (my mother's sister's husband), an internationally known expert in group process and psychotherapy, has been a caring mentor and important influence. Saul, a holocaust survivor, has helped me to see the powerful interplay of individual and collective forces in every aspect of human life.

An event that occurred at the beginning of my first year in medical school reified the intellectual (read ineffectual)/activist dichotomy I had established in my mind. The class that entered Harvard Medical School in September 1951 included about 45% Jewish students, many of whom had graduated from Harvard College. Evidently, whatever quotas there had been for admitting Jewish students to the medical school had been quite completely relaxed. It quickly became established that we — the Jewish students — were regarded by the "jocks" among the gentile students, who included several outstanding college football players, as eggheads if not wimps, even though Philip Isenberg, who had just been captain of the Harvard football team, was a member of our class.

So, to establish our athletic prowess and assert our masculine dignity, we, the Jewish students, did something that would probably be regarded now as too politically incorrect to be even contemplated. We challenged the gentile students to a softball game, to be played in the field behind the student dormitory (long since replaced by the Boston English High School building and parking lot). The outcome of the game, which went on until dusk, did not really matter. It all ended good humoredly in a tie. We Jewish intellectuals, from my distorted point of view, had certainly proved our activist credentials.

Then there is the matter of psychology. From childhood — age 12 sticks in my mind — I was searching out books in my elementary school library (it was a progressive school: Lincoln, later Horace Mann Lincoln, founded on the John Dewey principle of learning by doing) on psychology. The curiosity was driven, I think, by the restless hurt I felt inside. Like all explorers of the inner life, I suppose, the drive was to find out about others in order to make sense of my own raging uncertainties. But there is a problem in psychology for any would-be activist. As Freud turned from his thwarted political ambitions to do the politicians one better by understanding their motivations, psychology by its very nature is about analysis, not action.

There is a built-in suspicion of action in psychoanalysis, and perhaps psychology generally, which the inescapably pejorative though sometimes accurate term "acting out" implies. Activism may follow analysis through deliberate choice as problems are identified in the outer world that impact peoples' lives. But action for a psychologist (or a psychoanalyst as I later became) is not, I think, as close to his or her professional tradition as for physicians. Perhaps this is why, finally, after considering social psychology, I chose to become a medical psychologist or psychiatrist rather than follow a more purely academic path.

There is more to be said, I think, about the relationship between wound and action, at least in my own life. Partly to heal the pain connected with early losses, especially the death of my biological mother at 8 months (my father blamed the surgeon for not attending promptly enough to the peritonitis that followed a ruptured appendix), I embarked on a course of psychoanalytic treatment during medical school. A second analysis would later be required as part of psychoanalytic training. I am deeply grateful for the caring and meticulous understanding that my analysts offered. But I have come to feel that this process is too remote, too distant, too analytic, to reach and repair the wounds that reside in the deeper levels of the psyche, especially those associated with the losses and wounds of infancy. Something more powerful, more experiential, is essential, I think, and I have been exploring alternative therapeutic methods in recent years.

But even the most powerfully healing therapeutic approaches do not necessarily translate into social action, although there are in some psychological traditions, especially those like Buddhism that have a strong spiritual base, an emphasis on service and caring for others as an essential part of the transformative process. Here also I came to feel, beginning in my 30s, that depth psychology by itself was too self-oriented and incomplete in its therapeutic approaches. Something more was needed, a giving to others, taking on, if not slaying, the collective dragons, the institutional pathogens, that often seemed to be as much the source of human misery as our historical interactions with hurtful or depriving individuals. Like 12-step work in AA, which follows the work of abstinence and repair in alcoholism with a commitment to community service, some effort to contribute to human well-being outside of one's immediate family I now believe is an essential dimension of the therapeutic process. Thus, social action and inner healing have become, for me, inseparably linked.

My youth seems to have been consumed with an endless credentialing. Get this or that "ticket" so that you can do what you *really* want to do later, as if one ever can fully know. College followed high school; medical school followed college; and various house officerships followed one another (internship, adult psychiatric residency, child psychiatry fellowship) in a sequence of relentless preparations broken only by two crucial years in Japan working as a psychiatrist in the U.S. Air Force. I think of how my children have taken time after high school before college, and after college before graduate school, to travel, to work and play, and to learn about themselves and the world. This was unthinkable to my career-minded family, where even the traditional college junior year abroad was considered an indulgence.

But why did I comply with this constriction of life and vision? I like to think that the 1950s and early 1960s were like that, but I believe now that there was also a failure of imagination, a fear of breaking with my subculture's program for fulfilling ambitions and acquiring prestige. Things could have happened then that were different. When I complained as a junior staff person to Jack Ewalt, my boss at the Massachusetts Mental Health Center, that I did not have enough time to spend with my family, he made it clear that the work (to go up the career ladder) came first, and I should make appointments, as he had done, to see my small children. Mercifully for children and parents, all that is changing now. Psychoanalytic training should have helped, but it didn't. For psychoanalysis contributes more to understanding than to liberation. It can point the way to the experiences needed for personal growth, but it can also instill a certain self-consciousness, an overemphasis on an obsessive kind of self-reflection.

One of the most challenging areas for psychology is the study of how identity both changes and remains the same throughout a person's lifetime. We can identify a kind of core, containing in my case a reformist zeal, a certain pleasure in shaking things up. Even as a psychiatry resident, I was trying to replace the inpatient services at the Massachusetts Mental Health Center (MMHC), formerly the Boston Psychopathic Hospital, with partial hospitalization programs. But what has changed, at least for me, has been the size of the playing field. The scope of what I have undertaken seems continuously to have widened. In my writings, and in more direct social action, I have always been trying in some way to change the way people see or define themselves — first as individuals, later in relation to other groups, and, most recently, within the cosmos itself.

In the fall of 1958, I went to Washington to speak with the consultant to the Surgeon General about where I might be assigned for the 2 years of obligatory military service that lay ahead — doctors could do that then. I had hoped to be assigned to a base near Boston so I could simultaneously pursue psychoanalytic training. Colonel Paul Eggertson would hear none of this. Wearing a colorful California-type print shirt, he showed me in his characteristic breezy manner a map of the world with pins stuck where the Air Force (I had chosen the Air Force because it seemed more romantic) had assignments for psychiatrists. He seemed determined to send me overseas whether I liked it or not. Wiesbaden in West Germany was the plum for career officers, and Wheeler in Libya was out for a Jew, which left France, England, and Japan. Eggertson had loved his tours of duty in Japan, and I should have suspected what was going to happen. If he insisted on sending me out of the country, I preferred England or France. My orders for Japan came a few months later. I believe now that Eggertson knew this would be good for me. If he is still living and ever reads this, I want him to know that he has my eternal gratitude.

I was married in July 1959 to Sally Stahl shortly before leaving for Japan, and the 2 years there were crucial for all that has followed. Tachikawa Air Force Hospital, 20 miles west of Tokyo, was the "tertiary care" (base) hospital for the Air Force and Army in the Far East. Although 1959–1961 was a period between wars, I learned about the stresses of service for young men, the ruthlessness of military institutions, and the emotional trauma of cultural displacement for men, women, and children. Above all, this was my first experience of living in a foreign culture, and I came to realize how profoundly ethnocentric my view of the world had become.

In some ways Japan was a 2-year honeymoon. Sally and I lived in part of a large, old Japanese-style house in the village of Akishima near the base, and my first son, who was born there, was treated by our Japanese helpers and other friends with the reverence that only this complex and contradictory people bestow on infants and small children. I learned enough Japanese to speak with my neighbors, and life in Akishima taught me how fanatically ethnocentric and ecologically destructive we Americans can be. My first lesson on that score came when I discovered to my horror that the energy load created by our electrical appliances and 60-watt light bulbs required that the entire village be rewired.

We returned to the United States in the summer of 1961 with our 15-month-old son Danny, whose irritability and diarrhea reflected his separation from Japan, especially from Fujimoto-san, our devoted housekeeper who had loved him as if he had been her own child. I soon began a child psychiatry residency at the Massachusetts Mental Health Center, followed later by training in child analysis. Work with children has, in a sense, kept me honest. Children can hold us closer to the worlds of myth and imagination. They invite us to get down on the floor with them and make it difficult for the therapist to escape into his head. Working with children clinically, like raising them, can keep our spontaneity alive. Children live in a world of feeling and action and remind us of the continuity of generations. It is often with the threats and possibilities for their futures in mind that we work to create a better world.

During my child psychiatry residency, with the encouragement of psychoanalyst Peter Knapp at the Boston Psychoanalytic Institute (where I began training in the fall of 1961), I undertook a study of children's nightmares, which led to several articles and my first book, *Nightmares and Human*

Conflict, first published in 1970.[2] Nightmares and night terrors, as I understand them now, are profound expressions of human vulnerability. They occur when the psyche is threatened both from within and without and reflect the struggle to confine the terrors of existence to the nighttime. When this is not possible, when the center does not hold, psychological fragmentation can occur, and, as Mark Twain once wrote, the fears of the night can become the madness of the day.

Some time in the fall of 1964, my brother-in-law, Sidney Ingbar, told me that Harvard Medical School, where I was now a junior faculty member, was developing an affiliation with the Cambridge City Hospital. This community facility, less than a mile from Harvard Square, had fallen on hard times and could not maintain the quality of its services in a metropolitan area where teaching hospitals were attracting the best-trained physicians, nurses, and other personnel. In response to initiatives of town physicians and Cambridge officials, the Medical School arranged with the hospital administration to assign full-time chiefs of medicine, surgery, and pediatrics to begin in the summer of 1965. These chiefs would report to "parent" department heads at the Boston City (then a Harvard teaching hospital) and Massachusetts General Hospitals. The school was acting out of a combination of motives. On the one hand, there was the opportunity to develop a model of community-based primary health care. At the same time it was embarrassing for the university to have a derelict city hospital virtually in its own neighborhood in an age of expanding academic medicine.

Feeling somewhat restless in my middle-management position in charge of an inpatient service at the Massachusetts Mental Health Center, then Harvard Medical School's central psychiatric teaching facility, I asked Sid Ingbar what was planned for psychiatry at Cambridge City Hospital. He was based at Boston City and was in on the initial planning, having been asked by his chief, Dr. Maxwell Finland, to be the first Harvard chief of medicine at the newly affiliated hospital (which he declined). Sid told me that psychiatry was under medicine at Cambridge, and we discussed the possibilities for developing unique mental health services based at the hospital. In a note to myself dated December 28, 1964, I wrote "virgin area — exciting." Over the next few months I had conversations with a number of people who were responsible for the development of the Cambridge affiliation and persuaded Jack Ewalt, my chief and chairman of the Harvard Department of Psychiatry, that he should form a direct affiliation with the Cambridge City Hospital and permit me to oversee the development of the services and teaching program there. He agreed, and residents began a rotation in Cambridge as consultants on the medical and surgical wards in the summer of 1966.

Federal laws passed in the framework of the 1963 Kennedy Mental Health Act provided funding for staffing and construction of mental health facilities throughout the United States. In order to be eligible for these funds, the states had to come up with plans that involved creating regions or "catchment areas" within which mental health and retardation programs would be developed. In 1965, the cities of Cambridge and Somerville, with a total population of nearly 200,000, were designated as one such catchment area. Community leaders in the two cities considered the possibility that the Cambridge City Hospital might become the central facility of a potentially outstanding community mental health center, affiliated with the Harvard Medical School through the Department of Psychiatry.

After 2 years of planning for mental health services in Cambridge and Somerville from the Massachusetts Mental Health Center, I moved in July 1967 into an office in the former nursing school that was once connected with the Cambridge City Hospital (renamed the Cambridge Hospital in the late 1960s to remove the onus of the word "City"). This seemed at the time like a lonely journey into a foreign jungle, for when it came to public psychiatry, Cambridge was a new frontier despite its proximity to Harvard and the many citizens in Cambridge and Somerville committed to the development of high-quality community services. At the same time, what made this opportunity so exciting was the chance to put together city, state, and private resources with the backing (if it could be secured) of Harvard Medical School to create a mental health service system that cared for all the citizens in our area, especially, as my dear late colleague and friend Lee Macht phrased it, "those unable to take care of themselves."

Those of us who worked together in the 1960s and 1970s to create the Department of Psychiatry at the Cambridge Hospital and the Cambridge/Somerville Mental Health and Retardation Center shared a vision, which seems still to endure despite the medicalization of psychiatry generally and the dehumanization of mental health systems in this country. It is hard, like anything deeply felt with which one's life has been intimately associated, to put this into words. It has something to do with holism and spirit, building an institutional system that combines the intellectual riches (the academic resources of Cambridge have been important for this effort) with a dedication, quite fierce at times, to serving others relatively selflessly.

Power has been important, especially for the enrollment of local, state, and national political leaders in the department and hospital's mission. But it has been power used in the context of love and service. It is striking to me after 30 years of association with the Cambridge Hospital that people with "big egos," who use their work too unthinkingly for personal ambition and advancement, or become trapped in hierarchical forms of professionalism, do not last there very long.

The Cambridge "system" has its ways, sometimes gentle, sometimes tough, of putting people out on the sidewalk with a one-way ticket home. The Cambridge Hospital straddles geographically and psychologically the junction of the city's town and gown communities. Perhaps it is the more than

350 years of working out this accommodation that has provided the background for the hospital's culture. For it seems to be those who can bridge the hard-edged, sometimes detached, requirements of the academic teaching hospital (albeit one primarily devoted to basic, hands-on services) and the rough and tumble directness of city and community life and relationships that appear to survive best in our setting.

Furthermore, psychiatry in the best sense means the capacity to suspend one's personal ambitions in order to be able to perceive and identify with the needs of others at both the individual and organizational levels. The success of the psychiatry department at the Cambridge Hospital has resulted, it seems to me, from just this quality. Our department, beginning with the work of its pioneers, has been appreciated in the city for its responsiveness to the community's needs and for the willingness of its members to put aside personal agendas in the service of a larger purpose.

In my leadership role, what I sought to help create was a structure that was truly sensitive to individual human needs within a caring institutional context. I wanted to develop a model for mental health services that placed the knowledge of neuroscience and psychopharmacology within a psychosocial, humanistic, and even spiritual context. My style of leadership — easier perhaps for others to define than for me — has been to enroll people in a shared vision of possibilities that stretch their imagination while at the same time encouraging maximum freedom and responsibility-taking within the limits of personal and organizational realities. This has applied to everyone from junior mental health workers or other paraprofessional levels to senior medical faculty.

The years 1967 to 1971, when we began our own psychiatric residency at the hospital, were heady years for those of us involved in developing the department and the Mental Health Center. It was an experiment in building neighborhood- and community-based services in an academic context that seems to have worked. The late 1960s was a time of crisis and opportunity for psychiatry in particular and Cambridge Hospital in general. I cannot acknowledge adequately the enormous contributions that so many dedicated people made to the development of the Cambridge and Somerville health system during those years, for the realization of organizational possibilities depends almost entirely on the commitment of individuals and the willingness of those people to submerge their private agendas within the context of a larger, shared purpose. I fear even to mention my colleagues and friends of those times lest I offend someone whose contribution was essential or vital but whose story does not intertwine quite so directly with my own.

Edward Khantzian, one of the residents in my training group at MMHC and a warm aristocrat of working-class Armenian background who has never lost the common touch, began to go to Cambridge Hospital at the beginning of 1966 to supervise the rotating residents and begin the development of consultation/liaison (CL) and emergency services. The late Peter Reilly moved with me to Cambridge in July 1967 as the first chief resident and helped to set limits with me to the services we could provide while planning for the future. My secretary and assistant, Patricia Carr, was the only other person who crossed the river with me to Cambridge that summer. The creative and supportive part she has played over three decades has been central to the whole enterprise. Robert Reid, who had pioneered child and community services in Cambridge since 1955, became the first director of the mental health center, while I was in charge of its clinical services. The trust he had built among citizens and community leaders throughout Cambridge was essential to the success of our work. Along with William Ackerly, who developed the Somerville Mental Health Center in the 1960s, we worked as a kind of trio in putting together the pieces of the larger Cambridge/Somerville Mental Health Center structure.

In the summer of 1968 I was joined at Cambridge Hospital by James Beck and Lee Macht, former trainees of mine at MMHC, both of whom had completed 2 years of a military service equivalent at the National Institute of Mental Health in Washington, and by Susan Miller (later Susan Miller Havens), who had been a student and staff nurse at MMHC. While still in her mid-20s she developed the psychiatric nursing services in Cambridge. Sue went on to obtain an Ed.D. at Harvard and has become a national leader and expert in the field of adoption studies, services, and policies. The savvy of Beck and Macht about the mental health grant process from the other side — Jim had actually worked in the federal office that awarded the grants and knew how to write applications for them — greatly facilitated the process by which Cambridge and Somerville were awarded a $900,000 staffing grant, the largest given up to that time to any area. This grant, which provided for inpatient, outpatient, partial hospitalization, emergency, alcohol, drug, child, mental retardation, and other basic services, went into effect in July 1969 after many community meetings and late night calls to key Cambridge and Somerville state legislators to be sure that the item was not deleted in the logrolling that still accompanies the political process.

The role of Lee Macht, after whom the former nursing school building that houses the psychiatry department offices (which now occupy more than three floors) was named after his death in 1981, can hardly be described. He was my closest colleague and ally in the struggles of the early years. There was nothing we did not talk over, and the combination of wisdom and caring that he brought to the clinical and political work of building the department was unique, especially in someone so young. Lee, along with many of the early founders of the department, including Bob Reid and Bill Ackerly, was a child psychiatrist, which probably contributed to the strong developmental, family, and neighborhood orientation of the organization. His specialty, however, was neighborhood psychiatry, the provision of services in the locations where people lived that took into account the local realities that affected people's lives. The extensive system of neighborhood health clinics connected with the Cambridge Hospital owes a good deal to Lee's influence.

Lee succeeded me as chairman of our department in 1977, and his sudden death in 1981 at age 43 of food aspiration connected with an omental anomaly (the omentum is a fibrous membrane that protects the organs of the upper and midabdomen) was a profoundly tragic episode in the history of the department and the hospital. The former nursing school that housed our department was modernized in a renovation program effected by Myron Belfer, who succeeded Lee as department chairman, and Michael Greene, his chief administrative assistant. The building was named in Lee's honor — the Lee B. Macht Community Health Center — in a ceremony presided over by Harvard's President Derek Bok and city officials. In addition to the psychiatry offices, the building now houses the administrative offices of the Cambridge Health Commissioner and the Departments of Medicine, Surgery and Pediatrics.

A central figure in the organization and development of health services in Cambridge was James B. Hartgering, who was recruited in November 1967 by Leona Baumgartner, a pioneer in American public health, to become Commissioner of a newly reorganized Department of Health and Hospitals. A former army colonel, Hartgering had been an advisor on health science matters to President Johnson. He was a hard-drinking, no-nonsense, bear of a man whose warm but gruff ways, abrasive at times, got the job done. When he resigned in 1974, remarried, and retired to Cape Cod to live with the secretary who had worked with him at the hospital, he left behind a well-functioning health system that has since become a national model of excellence in service to its community.

I liked Jim Hartgering and worked well with him. Soon after we met, the Commissioner decided, as he wrote in a letter of recommendation for my professorial promotion in 1970, that I was "the person most committed to stabilizing the hospital and its internal programs." As a result, we met frequently one on one or with others to address the endless succession of town–gown, academic, personality, organizational systems, and other administrative problems that were constantly surfacing. Although there is no question that psychiatry benefited from my close relationship with Hartgering, which was itself subjected to criticism and even attack by jealous individuals at times, he had always seen the importance of strong mental health services in a complex and varied community such as Cambridge. My greatest challenge was to remain as disinterested and nonpartisan as humanly possible in addressing non-psychiatric problems with the Commissioner, especially those involving the Department of Medicine, while at the same time functioning as head of our department.

With Hartgering's insistence, we opened, in September 1968, an 11-bed inpatient psychiatric service, the hospital's first, on the fifth floor next to a self-care unit in the newly opened main building of the hospital. In retrospect, this may have been a bit premature. We did not yet have federal and state funding, and our thin staff was dependent on city money. Safety precautions were incomplete, and we paid for this when a Harvard law student, recently hospitalized for depression, swallowed some Clinitest tablets that a diabetic self-care patient was using to monitor her urine for glucose and ketones, pried open an inadequately secured window, and dropped himself out, landing on a grassy ledge three floors below. The patient survived the fall with broken vertebrae, but the Clinitest tablets contained lye, which eroded through his gastrointestinal system, causing a severe peritonitis from which he finally died at the Massachusetts General Hospital 4 weeks later.

The young man's father, who turned out to be a well-connected, wealthy lawyer, sued the psychiatric staff at the hospital. The suit turned out to be a kind of trial for the new service from which we learned many lessons, especially the importance of working closely with bereaved family members after a suicide, which I and other staff members, responding to bad advice, had failed to do. The case was finally settled out of court in 1975.

A dramatic experience in learning to cover my flanks occurred in November 1968, when Dr. Hartgering invited me to a meeting of the Cambridge City Council to address neighborhood anxieties about the new inpatient and community psychiatric services. Despite the fact that the law student was lingering near death at MGH, I was proud and cocky as I listed the benefits of the new unit, especially in preventing patients from having to go to the Westborough State Hospital, 35 miles to the west, which had been the previous fate of the mentally ill in Cambridge and Somerville. I had arranged for Mayor Walter Sullivan, an influential figure in Cambridge, to speak of how pleased one of his constituents had been with the new service, which made a strong impression at the meeting.

I was spiking, effectively I thought, the rumors flying around about what our unsavory patients were doing to themselves or to others in the hospital neighborhood. Things were, indeed, going well, and the Commissioner was pleased until veteran Councilor Alfred Vellucci, known for his ability to go to the heart of any matter, especially when it involved skewering someone or something connected with Harvard, bellowed at me, "Dr. Mack, I heard that a patient of yours jumped out the window of the fifth floor of the hospital. Was that a rumor?" Realizing my balloon was burst, I answered meekly that no, Councilor, that was not a rumor but a fact and explained the matter as best I could. Vellucci would bellow at me many more times in the years to come, but he and his son, Al Jr., who is still very actively involved in the hospital's administration, became among our strongest allies. Although politically conservative, Vellucci's caring for the welfare of his constituents is legendary, and we, in turn, were able from time to time to provide support as needed to members of his extensive family. That has been, always, the Cambridge way. In 1977, after I won a Pulitzer Prize for a biography of T. E. Lawrence,[3] Vellucci, who was then Mayor, arranged a ceremony at City Hall in which I was made an honorary citizen of the City of Cambridge.

The development of the Psychiatry Division, which did not become separated from Medicine as a distinct department until 1969, depended largely on the fate of the hospital itself and, above all, on the stability of the Department of Medicine. Indeed, the success or failure of the entire Harvard affiliation, and, in turn, the future of the hospital and its associated health system depended on the medical service — which is probably true for any hospital. It is not surprising then that the most severe crisis that the hospital has undergone in my 30 years of association with it occurred following the resignation in 1968 of Dr. George Nichols, the first permanent medical chief, whose Yankee patrician ways did not mingle well with the give and take of Cambridge's multiethnic health politics.

The responsibility for selecting Dr. Nichols' successor resided with Dr. James Jandl, an internationally renowned hematologist and the hand-picked successor, as head of Harvard's Boston City Hospital service, of the legendary medical giant William Castle. Jandl was tailor-made not to be able to do this job. Research and specialty oriented himself, he could not really value the primary care mission of the hospital.

As the months went by, the crisis deepened. Senior internists came over from the Boston City Hospital for 1-month stints as acting chiefs of medicine at Cambridge. Supervision of medical house officers became thinner and thinner as senior medical physicians withdrew from the leaderless department. This had the effect of leading the other Harvard Chiefs of Medicine (at the Massachusetts General, Peter Bent Brigham, and Beth Israel Hospitals) to threaten to withdraw their rotating residents on whom the hospital's basic care depended. Even Jandl threatened to withdraw his own residents. The chiefs gave the end of 1969 as a deadline for Cambridge to obtain a chief of medicine, or they would withdraw the residents. But this created an impossible catch-22 situation, as finding a chief of medicine was the responsibility of one of Harvard's medical chiefs, Dr. Jandl.

The end of December 1969 was a dark time. The Commissioner, Sid Ingbar (who, partly as a favor to me, had signed on for a longer rotation as acting chief at Cambridge), and I were able to persuade Dean Robert Ebert, who was unable to control his feudal medical chiefs, to order them at least to continue the residents until June 1970. The crisis was temporarily averted, but as the spring of the year arrived, this deadline loomed large, and something had to be done.

An opportunity to resolve the problem presented itself in May. Sid Ingbar, again in cooperation with me, agreed, at Dean Ebert's request, to take over the chairmanship of the search committee for Dr. Nichols' successor, as by this time it was clear to everyone involved that Dr. Jandl could not do the job. But there remained the impossible obstacle that any chief would still have to report to Jandl, and Dean Ebert simply did not feel he had the power to change the lines of affiliation. The break came when Dr. John Knowles, then Director of the Massachusetts General Hospital, offered to take over the administration of the entire Cambridge Hospital, including the Department of Medicine.

Such a loss of autonomy was unthinkable to the City of Cambridge and all of us involved with the hospital. But we did not tell Knowles that. Instead, we used his grandiose offer (highly ambitious and able, Knowles would later become president of the Rockefeller Foundation) as an opportunity to resolve our smaller, more specific problem. Such an offer could be interpreted as creating a policy crisis that could be dealt with only at the highest level. Tucking the Cambridge Hospital into MGH, after all, was a matter that could only be decided by the City Government and, appropriately, with the participation of Harvard's highest official, its President. So Commissioner Hartgering discussed the matter with Dean Ebert, who invited Harvard's mild-mannered President, Nathan Pusey, soon to leave office, to a meeting in the hospital cafeteria. This historic gathering took place on May 26, 1970. It was chaired by the commissioner and was also attended by the City Manager of Cambridge, (then) Mayor Vellucci, members of the Cambridge City Council, Dean Ebert, all the Harvard chiefs of medicine, John Knowles, and all of the Cambridge department heads.

The first 2 hours of the meeting were spent in reviewing in detail the history of the problem and the looming catastrophe, as the medical residents were scheduled to depart at the end of June. As it became clear to Dr. Knowles that the real agenda for the meeting was not his proposal to take over the hospital but the problem of breaking the impasse in medicine, he gracefully subsided. The meeting came to a definitive conclusion when President Pusey turned to Dean Ebert and, in his soft voice, instructed him, according to my notes (I took virtually verbatim notes, which, when typed up, ran to 7½ pages, single spaced), "to call a meeting of the chiefs of the Departments of Medicine with Dr. Ingbar, the Dean, and Dr. Lee [Sidney Lee, Associate Dean for Hospitals] in order to resolve the problem of obtaining a chief [of medicine for Cambridge]."

For me this was the turning point, a decisive moment in the hospital's history, for it enabled a workable restructuring of the search process to occur and placed on record Harvard's commitment at the highest level to support the hospital in a time of major crisis. No crisis of this magnitude has occurred in the intervening 25 years, in part, perhaps, because of the implicit availability of the power of Harvard's President and his willingness to get involved if things got bad enough at this sensitive hot spot of town–gown relationships in the university's backyard.

President Pusey's words empowered Dean Ebert to remove the Cambridge Hospital's Department of Medicine from
Dr. Jandl's jurisdiction. Within a few weeks Arnold Weinberg,
a brilliant, charismatic infectious disease specialist, was selected by Dr. Ingbar's committee to be Chief of Medicine.
During his 5 years at Cambridge, Weinberg laid the groundwork for a first-rate department of medicine. Alcohol services
(administered jointly by medicine and psychiatry) and other
essential mental health programs could then grow rapidly.

Over the last 25 years the Department of Psychiatry at
the Cambridge Hospital has been fulfilling its potential as
one of the outstanding psychosocially and humanistically oriented departments in the country. Residency positions with
Dr. Leston Havens as residency training director are highly
coveted, as are training slots in psychology, social work, and
nursing. The medical student rotations under Dr. Alfred Mar-
gulies' leadership receive top ratings. The department has
benefited from the able leadership, after Lee Macht's death,
of Myron Belfer, Malkah Notman, and Deborah Moran. Meanwhile, the hospital itself has emerged as one of most distinguished community service institutions in the United States,
especially under the wise and strong guidance of its present
administrator, John O'Brien. In 1993 it won the prestigious
Foster McGaw award for excellence in community service, a
$75,000 prize that recognized the vast array of people-sensi-
tive hospital- and neighborhood-based services. These include
health care for the homeless, a multidisciplinary AIDS program, school-based child and teen-age health centers, house
calls for the homebound elderly, and linguistic minority programs as well, of course, as various drug, alcohol, and mental
health services.

For me the Cambridge Hospital experience lies at the
core of my work as a physician. All that I have done since
the pioneering years of the late 1960s and early 1970s has
derived, at least in part, from what I learned in the trenches
of the Cambridge health system. These have been simple

principles that begin with community service and the understanding of the psychological and political forces operating in
group systems. In any planning process, I have discovered,
it is essential to identify and include all those who have a
stake in the outcome. People can share in a vision if they
are able to participate in its fulfillment. Individuals who feel
excluded will undermine what you are trying to achieve, even
when they do not consciously know or acknowledge that they
are doing so. A common ground of shared interest can almost
always be found, as I discovered with the McGovern family
of obstetricians. The McGoverns — the late Philip Sr. and his
sons Philip Jr., head of obstetrics at the Hospital, and Arthur
— had delivered a good proportion of the babies of Cambridge
over several decades. Initially skeptical about our services,
they recognized the value they had for their patients and the
community and became among our staunchest allies, opening
political doors we could not have passed through on our own.

Another principle concerns the use of power. As physicians, we are always engaged in power relations of one kind
of another, although we may not recognize this. At the same
time, we have little understanding and surely no training
about how power works or how to use it. For me this was a
big part of the learning on the job in Cambridge. I found
that I had to discover where decision-making power resided
in the city, state, medical school, and other institutions involved in Cambridge/Somerville health care, find a way to
communicate with these individuals, and bring them into an
evolving shared vision of an exemplary health care system.
The use of power can be frightening, especially when we deny
that we are dealing with it. But this fear generally relates
to the egoistic aspect, to relating the project to oneself. The
best antidote, I have learned, for this anxiety, which can enable one to proceed, is the realization that we are simply
playing a role that is a vehicle for serving a larger purpose.

The stakes often seemed high during the years when the
Harvard affiliation in Cambridge was becoming established,

and I found myself deeply identified with the project and the success of the venture. This made for some highly worrisome times, especially when one or another vital program was threatened because of competing economic and political priorities. I began this work in the relatively prosperous times for mental health of the 1960s. I think I would have found the economic and bureaucratic savaging of mental health care since the 1970s personally intolerable and admire the administrators who endured and prevailed in these difficult times.

My work in Cambridge came to parallel a strong interest in the life and psychology of T. E. Lawrence ("Lawrence of Arabia"). In September 1963, when Sally was 8 months pregnant with our third son, Tony, we went to see the film *Lawrence of Arabia*. We came late and ended up in the second balcony. The theater was hot, the desert scenes were hot, and Sally was very hot. But I was excited by the character of Lawrence despite the inevitable Hollywood distortions (T. E. Lawrence, for instance, was 5 feet 4 and Peter O'Toole well over 6 feet). Until then Lawrence had been for me a romantic, heroic figure, vaguely tainted with perversion. The film stimulated me to learn more about him, for he seemed to embody the tension between inner purpose and action and the possibility that an individual might live out a creative vision on the world's stage. I read everything that I could lay my hands on about Lawrence and wrote to his two then-living brothers to see if they would talk with me about him if I came to England. This led to interviews in 1964 with T. E.'s older brother, Robert, in Dorset and youngest brother, Arnold, in London. Two other brothers were killed in World War I.

Arnold, an archeologist as T. E. had been, was only 64 when I met him. He became a lively, witty, and helpful collaborator who grasped well my various notions about his brother's psychology and motivation. It was he, more than anyone else, who made the book possible, for he led me to many unpublished sources, including embargoed family documents, as well as to family friends, service companions, and a variety of other friends and colleagues of his famous brother. My research was a kind of treasure hunt in search of people and papers that took me all over the British isles, to Majorca (to interview Robert Graves, who wrote, after Lowell Thomas's popular potboiler, the first real biography of Lawrence), and, of course, to the Middle East, where I was still able to find Bedouin Arabs who had fought with Lawrence during the years of the Arab Revolt.

I learned several important things in this study, which was published, finally, in 1976 as a book, *A Prince of Our Disorder: The Life of T. E. Lawrence,*[3] that won a Pulitzer Prize for biography. First, I developed a strong distrust of popular representations of controversial figures. For Lawrence was far from being just a romantic impostor, as he was often described. Rather he turned out to be, for me, a complex figure who, despite a number of psychological problems, was the principal force in galvanizing and supporting the Arab revolt against Turkey and had a fair amount to do with shaping the map of the contemporary Middle East. Second, I developed a profound respect for what a human being can do with, or in spite of, a great deal of personal conflict and psychopathology if an avenue for individual personal expression, including political involvement and action, is available. Indeed, I have become forever deeply suspicious of any psychological analysis that looks only at pathology and overlooks the creative enactment that a person has pursued in his world.

Finally, from Lawrence himself, I learned about working as a stranger in a community or culture that is not one's own. In his case, his illegitimacy and the marginality of his family background and birth contributed to the fluidity of identity that may be a prerequisite of special creativity in this area. My search for T. E. Lawrence in Europe and the Middle East seemed to parallel my own more modest work in Cambridge, where I often felt like, and was, pretty much of an outsider, at least for many years.

Lawrence's "Twenty-Seven Articles,"[4] published during the war among his dispatches from the Middle East, set down basic principles for working with his Arab allies. They contain many psychological principles of leadership that apply when one is not directly in charge but must work through others in positions of authority, as was true for him among the Arab chieftains and, of course, for me in Cambridge. In Article 8, for example, he wrote,

> Your ideal position is when you are present and not noticed. Do not be too intimate, too prominent, or too earnest. Avoid being identified too long or too often with any tribal sheikh, even if C/O of the expedition. To do your work you must be above jealousies, and you lose prestige if you are associated with a tribe or clan and its inevitable feuds. (p. 464)

In 1966, when I was in the early stages of the Lawrence project, I consulted L. Carl Brown, who was then a young professor of political science at Harvard specializing in the Middle East, about some of the things I needed to know if I were to venture into the history and politics of that tortured region. Six years later, by which time Carl had moved to Princeton, he invited me to talk about Lawrence at a huge international conference he was planning on the psychology of the Middle East. The conference, which took place in May 1973, was followed by several smaller meetings at Princeton that addressed specifically the psychopolitics of the Arab–Israeli conflict. At these meetings I met psychiatrists William Davidson, Rita Rogers, and Vamik Volkan and foreign service officer Joseph Montville, who were engaged in looking at the emotional (we rather neglected the spiritual elements in those secular days) forces that were driving the Middle East conflict.

Over the next 8 years I participated with Egyptians, Palestinians, and other Arabs, Israelis, and Americans (including prominent American Jewish leaders) at many conferences and problem-solving workshops in the United States, Europe, and the Middle East. The purpose of these meetings, some of which were held under the auspices of the American Psychiatric Association, was twofold: to bring together unofficially representative protagonists of parties to the Arab–Israeli conflict in a safe setting who might otherwise be prevented from meeting by the political realities of the conflict (Montville has called this process "track II" diplomacy to distinguish it from official or "track I" diplomatic relationships); and to evolve a body of analytic principles that might be applied usefully in the amelioration of this and other ethnonational conflicts. Interactive conflict resolution is a growing field whose recognized value has not been matched by the hoped-for results, primarily because leaders determined to exploit for personal and nationalistic ends the historic hurts in their geographic regions have often been unwilling to permit the conciliatory principles of track II diplomacy to play a significant part in the political process.

My participation in the Middle East peace process involved me in a number of private, behind-the-scenes efforts to communicate between parties to the conflict. One of these involved a meeting with Yassir Arafat in Beirut in April 1980, arranged by Walid Khalidi, a Palestinian professor and leader who had become a friend at Harvard. Beirut was then in the midst of the anguish of its prolonged civil war. I had been invited to speak about Lawrence and related matters at the American University of Beirut (AUB) and to consult to the dean of the AUB medical school, who was trying, despite the wartime conditions, to improve the psychiatry department.

I was picked up at my hotel by armed Palestinians at night, taken through the darkened city and various checkpoints to a home in the Beirut district of one of Arafat's friends, where the meeting, which included other Palestinian leaders, would take place. The "Chairman," also referred to by those close to him as the "Old Man," arrived shortly after I did. Of relatively small stature, Arafat wore army clothes and a black-and-white *kaffiya* and showed the thin beard that is familiar to us. In my notes right after the meeting, I wrote, "He is a bit paunchy and yet there is a sympathetic quality to the man, a kind of directness. He meets you eye to eye, and you feel a determination and a clarity of mind."

The meeting, which lasted several hours, was concerned with a detailed review of the facts of the conflict, the legacy of resolutions proferred, neglected, or broken, his personal grief over the Palestinian diaspora and losses sustained in the conflict (Hammami, one of Arafat's closest associates, had just been murdered by Iraqi extremists), and the deep sadness on all of our parts that greater trust and reason had not prevailed. Specifically, Arafat hoped that I would convey to the American Jewish leaders with whom I was then in contact his willingness to settle for a Palestinian homeland on the West Bank and Gaza and to do my part in dispelling the notion that such a step would be but the first stage in taking over the whole of Palestine, i.e., the destruction of Israel. As I left, there were about a half-dozen armed PLO gunmen outside the apartment whom I had not noticed before. The same car was waiting, and I was driven efficiently back to my hotel.

Ethnonationalism serves a wealth of deep individual and collective needs, beginning with survival but including as well the desire to belong to a body or entity larger than oneself and the sense of positive or negative self-esteem, power or powerlessness, that accompanies the fate of one's ethnic group or nation. But at root, ethnonationalism is a matter of identity — of mistaken identity in my view. The fact that many millions of people have died for ethnonational causes, voluntarily or at the hands of leaders who have manipulated their minds, coerced their participation in the slaughter of nationalistic wars, or murdered them outright with the justification of one or another genocidal ideology is perhaps the lead story of the century now coming to a close. The only way to avoid the final omnicidal convulsion, it seems to me, would be to discover a different, expanded, human identity, what the Cherokee Nation has called our "original instructions." This would involve a redefinition of who we are at a human level, a species that has unique ethnonational subgroups within it perhaps, but one that is connected fully to all human groups on a planet in which we discover ourselves to be, once again, connected spiritually and nondenominationally at a cosmic level.

At one of the Princeton meetings in November 1973, I met Rita Rogers, a child psychiatrist from California, who was there to present a paper on David Ben-Gurion, one of the founders of the state of Israel. Born Rita Stenzler, she grew up in the town of Radauti in the province of Bukovina in northern Romania. Her parents were living in Haifa in 1973, and she had made frequent trips to visit them. Her most recent trip had been a mission of mercy to tend the wounded of the recent October or "*Yom Kippur*" war, where she found in a Haifa hospital among the injured men the as yet to be identified son of one of her friends who, unable to speak until he had recovered from surgery, was convalescing from a shrapnel wound to his head. I was impressed then with Rita's determination and courage. As we became friends over the next few years through our common efforts as psychiatrists addressing the psychological aspects of ethnonational conflict, she told me stories of her idyllic *haute bourgeois* childhood in Romania, the years with her family in a Romanian/German concentration camp, and the odyssey of her escapes from several communist regimes in the years after the war.

When I was asked in 1979 if I would contribute to the Harvard/Radcliffe biography series on American women, I thought I would like to write about Rita,[5] if she would qualify as an American, since she was 28 when she came here in 1953 to train in psychiatry. Deane Lord, director of the Harvard News Office, and Merloyd Lawrence of Addison-Wesley publishers, were in charge of the series and agreed to my proposal. Rita's and my researches together in the early 1980s took us to the Ukraine, Prague, Vienna, and, of course, the Bukovina — the places that had figured prominently in her life. We found the tragic remnants of the decimated Jewish communities of Eastern Europe, and yet Rita's story became as much one of transformation and community as of tragedy and suffering, although there was so much of both. For she had been fortunate and, through her wiles and strengths had been able to save her family and to emerge from the war and her years of flight relatively unscarred.

Rita's life became for me an example of the triumphant human spirit, of the possibility of transcending malignant ideologies without bitterness. She had become a leading figure in political psychology, translating her personal experiences into public commitment. Her personal example, together with her writings, bear witness to the possibility that destructive human divisions, what Erik Erikson has called pseudospeciation, can be overcome and that a shared human destiny may yet be discovered.

Of the many stories that we shared, one seems to capture best for me what my collaboration with Rita was really about. In June 1981, we brought with us to Eastern Europe her daughter Sheila, now an eminent young journalist, and my son Kenneth, now studying international relations at Columbia University, then respectively 20 and 19. On a train from Bucharest to Vinnitsa in the Ukraine, from which we were to go on to Mogilev Podolsky where the camp had been, we were awakened at the Soviet (Moldavian) border town of Ungheni in our four-person couchette at 4 AM — this kind of thing always seems to occur at 4 AM in Eastern Europe — by three or four customs officers. The man in charge wore a gray civilian suit and spoke English. The others wore khaki military-looking uniforms and did not say much. We had been bumped off the train on which we had originally been booked and transferred to this train, so evidently they did not have us on any list. Suspicious and confused about the purposes of four people, including an unmarried man and woman, traveling with passports under two names, the man in the gray suit instructed the other officials to dump all of our tape recording and camera equipment into several bags, which they removed from the train.

Rita, remembering her anxious year as a nomad in Bessarabia and northern Bukovina (taken by Stalin in a 1940 pact with Hitler and reclaimed in 1944) after liberation of the camp in April 1944, was afraid to reveal her history to Soviet officials and insisted that I represent our group and declare our purpose to be "tourism." This story did not go down at all with the man in the gray suit, who interrogated me in the corridor of the sleeping car as Sheila, Ken, and Rita remained in the couchette. He wanted to know how Rita and I had met, the kind of "medical" work we were doing in the Soviet Union, and the real purpose of this visit. The situation grew increasingly tense, for it was clear to him that tourists did not travel this way.

By the time of this trip I had become active in Physicians for Social Responsibility (PSR) and the physicians' antinuclear movement, but Rita had warned me not to talk about that because of the political aspects. Our plight on the train, however, seemed rather grim to me, so I decided to take a risk. I asked the man if he had heard of the physicians anti-nuclear movement and particularly of International Physicians for the Prevention of Nuclear War (IPPNW), whose first congress had recently been held at Airlee House in Virginia, an hour outside of Washington, D.C. I knew that the Soviet copresident of IPPNW, the eminent Russian cardiologist Evgeny Chazov, had spoken extensively after the congress on Soviet television about the dangers of nuclear war, the necessity of prevention, and the warm collaboration that was developing between the Soviet and American representatives when he indicated his familiarity with IPPNW. I told my interrogator that not only had I attended this congress, but I had sat at Dr. Chazov's table and given a toast for peace with vodka brought by our

Soviet friends. Immediately the man's demeanor changed, for evidently he had seen and heard Chazov on Soviet television. "You drank vodka with Dr. Chazov?!" he exclaimed warmly and enthusiastically. "That's wonderful!"

He told me then that everything would be fine. We were to go into the station building for some routine formalities, consisting, as it turned out, of brief questioning by another customs official, after which we were taken back to the train and our belongings promptly restored to us. Needless to say, Sheila and Ken had been wondering if they would see their parents again, and, as the train got under way again, I had to explain to Rita as well what had happened, for there had been no chance to tell her in the station. For me this experience was a sharp lesson in the necessity of being able to disobey instructions (in this case Rita's) when necessary. But more importantly, the incident testified to the vital importance of human connection and warmth, which alcohol has often facilitated, for transcending the dangerous separations that borders and boundaries create artificially between human beings.

In 1977, social psychiatrist Perry Ottenberg asked me to join a task force he was organizing under the American Psychiatric Association to examine what was then euphemistically called the "Psychosocial Aspects of Nuclear Advances." Also included in the group were Jerome Frank, a pioneer in our profession in looking at the destructive human forces that were driving the nuclear arms race, and child psychiatrist William Beardslee, with whom I would collaborate over the next few years in a number of studies of the impact of the threat of nuclear war on children and adolescents. Rita Rogers was its chairperson. In addition to examining the effect of the arms race on children, the task force also considered the psychology of the Soviet–American relationship, nuclear terrorism, and the emotional fallout from the 1979 accident at the Three-Mile Island nuclear power plant in Pennsylvania.

At the end of the 1970s my oldest son Daniel, who was then a student at Berkeley, was taking part in demonstrations against the Diablo Canyon nuclear power plant in California, and I remember saying to him that the nuclear arms race represented an infinitely greater threat to life than nuclear energy. His reply was telling, for he said that the political and military structure and secrecy surrounding the creation and deployment of nuclear weapons made that world seemingly impenetrable. It was precisely the political and psychological penetration of the nuclear-weapons-creating structure that was the principal enterprise of the physicians antinuclear movement, led by cardiologist Bernard Lown, the American copresident of IPPNW, and pediatrician Helen Caldicott, president of its American component, Physicians for Social Responsibility (PSR), which reached its peak effectiveness in the early 1980s in response to the escalation of the threat of nuclear war in the early years of the Reagan administration.

Our message through PSR, delivered in countless articles and major symposia around the country, was a simple but telling one: an actual nuclear "exchange" (one of the many euphemisms used to lull us into obliviousness in relation to the actualities of the nuclear threat) would bring destruction of human life on such a scale that no realistic medical response was possible. The only sane approach was prevention, we said, but that, of course, meant effective deescalation of the confrontation between the United States and the U.S.S.R. So, inevitably and, I thought, rather reluctantly, the leaders of the physicians' movement were drawn into the political arena, and our work received major media attention. Dr. Caldicott met with President Reagan, and Dr. Lown formed a positive relationship with Mikhael Gorbachev when he came into office in 1985.

Needless to say, all this was not well received by the conservatives in the White House and Congress, who challenged our legitimate right as physicians to become involved in political and military policy matters. Perhaps the most important outcome of the physicians' antinuclear movement, outside of whatever contribution it may have made to the reduction of the nuclear threat, was the clear establishment of the fact that the nuclear weapons problem was not the preserve of a secret government, scientific, and military elite. It was, rather, a crisis of human identity, an outcome of extreme ideological passion and conflicting nationalisms, a fundamental impasse in the ordering of group relationships on the planet. It was, therefore, a matter that was then, and remains, every citizen's responsibility.

At its peak in the early to mid-1980s PSR had 40,000 physician and nonphysician members, and IPPNW reported that physician participation in the more than 50 nations who were represented in its international congresses reached the hundreds of thousands. In 1985, IPPNW was awarded the Nobel Peace Prize for its work in reducing the threat of nuclear war. At the "heart" of this organization was the longstanding personal relationship of two cardiologists, Bernard Lown and Evgeny Chazov. Their vision of peace had grown out of a friendship cultivated in the course of many meetings at medical conferences in the years before they thought of starting IPPNW in 1980. My own work in PSR and IPPNW was focused on the emotional impact of the nuclear weapon competition and the threat of nuclear annihilation on children and adolescents and later on the psychosocial and psychospiritual roots of the arms race itself.

In October 1980, Rita Rogers invited Jack Ruina, an MIT professor of electrical engineering who had worked on defensive ballistic missile systems, to consult with our task force. Ruina made no secret of the fact that he considered the arms race to be irrational at its core. Hearing this from someone who had, himself, been one of the nuclear insiders, a group that social scientist Carol Cohn called "defense intellectuals,"[6] emboldened the task force, and me especially, to look at more fundamental psychosocial causes of the nuclear weapons competition. With Ruina's encouragement and contacts he and colleagues of mine at the Kennedy School of Government of Harvard provided, I was able to interview nuclear weapons decision makers in the Congress and executive branches of government, the weapons labs, and private industry. These included Robert McNamara, Robert McFarland, David Jones (former Chairman of the Joint Chiefs of Staff), Jimmy Carter, and Edward Teller. The purpose of the study,[7] which was originally to have included Soviet weapons makers, was to understand how each of these men understood his role in the nuclear weapons acquisition or policy process in order to reveal how the nuclear war system as a whole was propelled.

What struck me most powerfully was the fragmented nature of responsibility in relation to the nuclear threat that permitted each individual to do his particular job with a minimum of actual belief in the Soviet menace. Even Jimmy Carter felt that his efforts to put into practice his own desire for a better relationship with the Soviet Union was curtailed by the Congress and his need to make so many compromises to achieve the most modest of his objectives. For a number of these individuals, professional responsibility and competence took precedence over the vast potential consequences of the project in which they were engaged.

Of the 20 bomb makers whom I interviewed, only Teller, whom I met with at the Cosmos Club in Washington in 1986, was a driven ideologue. But perhaps it only required a few such men to provide the emotional fire and evoke the fear that propelled the competition on the American side. Teller's demonization of the Soviet Union, which was fused in his mind with the Nazi regime and the Holocaust, was unquestioning and, it seemed to me, quite irrational. When I asked him if he really believed that his invention, the Strategic Defense Initiative (SDI or "Star Wars"), could really work, he replied that it might save the State of Israel. The study taught me above all the danger of technocratic expertise and its associated fragmentation of responsibility in a world filled with instruments of mass destruction, what I have called "malignant professionalism."[8]

Studies conducted by Beardslee, me and others of children's fears of nuclear war, though methodologically flawed, touched a raw nerve in the culture and were used politically by Caldicott and the media. Headlines such as "Your Children Are Afraid" were blazoned across the country in the early 1980s, and letters of children to President Reagan led him to say in a November 1982 speech how troubled he was to learn of the fears and nightmares of children related to the nuclear threat, which seemed to be a factor in beginning his initiatives toward Soviet leaders. In 1984, I testified about this work before the House of Representatives Committee on Children and Families. The political impact of the not surprising finding that children and adolescents in this and other countries ranked high among their worries the possibility that they would not have a future because of the danger of nuclear war lay in the fact that the arms buildup was failing in its fundamental purpose — the provision of security, which is, at its root, a subjective, emotional matter. Furthermore, children and adolescents, when interviewed, would inevitably cut through the adult denial, euphemisms, and acronyms by speaking of burned bodies, mass death, and wasted landscapes.

In the fall of 1981, following the lead of the city of Cambridge, my son Kenneth decided to spearhead a campaign to provide truthful information about the realities of nuclear war for his home town of Brookline to counter the lying sanitization contained in the civil defense plan that was then being circulated by the federal government. This resulted in the publication of a booklet that Ken wrote with a little help from his parents and consultation from several experts; Ken had to raise private funds in order to have it widely distributed (unlike Cambridge, which had paid for its own pamphlet).

At a meeting of the Brookline Selectmen in January 1982, at which Ken's proposal was to be discussed, I met

Brookline teacher and assistant principal Roberta Snow, who had recently founded Educators for Social Responsibility in order to create curricula for schools that would provide solid information about the realities of nuclear war, the arms race, and the Soviet Union itself. Bobbi and I became comrades in arms, and together with psychiatrists Robert Jay Lifton, Eric Chivian (who had helped to found IPPNW), Richard Chasin, and William Beardslee and theologian Dorothy Austin, founded the Center for Psychological Studies in the Nuclear Age (later called the Center for Psychology and Social Change). The purpose of the Center, which is affiliated with the Harvard Medical School through the Department of Psychiatry at the Cambridge Hospital, has been to conduct studies and provide public education about the psychological and spiritual forces that underlie human behaviors that are destructive on a mass scale. As the immediacy of the nuclear threat has lessened with the end of the cold war, the Center's focus has shifted to the problems of ethnonationalism, corporate responsibility, and environmental destruction.

In the early 1980s the concentration of my psychopolitical interests shifted from the Middle East to the U.S.–Soviet relationship and its role in driving the nuclear weapons competition. To be politically effective in this dialogue it was not sufficient to underscore the demonization and dehumanization of the other side, whose irrationality and one-sidedness had become quite apparent to sensitive people by the early 1980s. It was necessary, in addition, to sort out the elements of real threat from those that were the product of our own political behavior or ideological distortions. But, above all, the task of the physicians and other groups working to reduce the nuclear threat was to make clear the collective arrogance, the primal madness, that underlay our and the Soviets' apparent willingness to destroy life on the planet as we know it over a difference of political perception and social values.

My work with Soviet colleagues through IPPNW, especially psychiatrist Marat Vartanian, led to several trips to the

Soviet Union on one or another "track II" mission. In the summer of 1983, with Vartanian's help, Eric Chivian was able to arrange an extensive series of interviews with boys and girls ranging in age from 11 to 16 at the Black Sea youth camp Orlyonok. To our surprise (we expected control and censorship), the children were allowed to speak freely with us and talked movingly, as American children had, of their fears of nuclear bombs and of not growing up. The film that we made with the help of a Russian film crew was shown on U.S. national television, including excerpts on *Nightline,* and in communities throughout the United States. It seemed to help to show the common humanity of young people and cut through the anti-Soviet stereotyping that was rampant in the United States at that time.

On my first trip to the Soviet Union in October 1979, my wife and I met in Tbilisi, Georgia, a young Russian, Mikhael Meylakh, then a romance language student in Leningrad. The conference, the first to be held in the Soviet Union on the unconscious and psychoanalysis since before the Stalin era, was organized, not surprisingly, by the independently minded Georgians. Meylakh, excited by the chance to meet Western psychiatrists and intellectuals, traveled to Tbilisi, where he came to symbolize for me the as yet unfulfilled opportunities for connection and exchange between American and Russian citizens. I was considering studying Russian, and Meylakh told me that he had a sister, Mirra, living in Boston who gave Russian lessons.

I failed to contact Mirra when I returned, and it was not until I had found myself traveling relatively frequently to Moscow that I looked her up in 1986. To my great dismay I discovered that Mikhael had been imprisoned for 3 years in a camp in the Ural mountains, where he was doing hard labor for no crime other than the exchanging of papers and ideas with Western colleagues and friends and his too great friendliness with people like me. Needless to say, I was outraged and joined the forces that were engaged in trying to get him and other political prisoners released by the Gorbachev regime that had come into power the previous year. The matter came to a head in January, 1987, when Richard Chasin and I were invited by Vartanian to attend an international conference in Moscow on forming partnerships and overcoming enmity.

At one point in the conference someone in the audience went on a one-sided tirade about the unjust American tendency to maintain an enemy image of the Soviet Union. I lost my temper and, as the television cameras rolled, gave a short speech, which I felt encouraged to continue by the approving gestures and faces of the journalists and other Soviets in the audience. I said that their country could go a long way toward changing its image in the United States by releasing unjustly imprisoned people, and I talked specifically about my friend Meylakh. The next morning Chasin and I were to meet with Vartanian, and I was afraid that I might have embarrassed our host, who had reached a high position by treading a fine line with several Soviet regimes. When he greeted us he said, pointing at the ceiling, "John, they liked what you did yesterday up there." Noticing his gesture I asked if he meant the Central Committee or God. "Here it is the same thing," he replied. A week or so later Meylakh was released along with a hundred or so other prisoners. I hope that my effort may have contributed to the outcome.

In June 1986, I was arrested with my wife and three sons, together with nearly 150 other people, for crossing the boundary into the nuclear weapons test site in Mercury, Nevada. Without testing, the nuclear arms race could not be maintained. This was my first experience with direct civil disobedience and came about as a result of the fact that the Reagan administration was continuing weapons testing despite a long Soviet moratorium. Daniel Ellsberg, who was one of the leaders of the action, also pointed out how troubled and disappointed I (and they) might feel if I chose, fearing for my reputation, a "support" instead of a more active role.

Ellsberg's words were instrumental in pushing me, psychologically and literally, over the edge.

Ken served 6 days in jail in Goldfield Nevada, and Sally 5 days in Tonopah. Danny, Tony, and I paid our fines and did not go to jail. The example of a whole family getting arrested received wide national media coverage, and Sally organized a group of families against nuclear testing, which resulted in bringing more people to the test site for protests and arrests in 1988 and 1989. It is difficult to know what contribution this nonviolent civil disobedience made to the eventual U.S. moratorium on nuclear testing in 1991. We were told that these actions, which at their peak involved many hundreds of arrests, were effective in influencing congressional opinion against nuclear testing.

I was criticized by a number of my colleagues for moving beyond the role of psychopolitical analysis to direct action. This would, they said, undermine my credibility as an objective academic and might interfere with the funding of studies related to the arms race that we were then undertaking. I thought deeply about this and came to the conclusion, after reading Thoreau and others, that such actions were altogether consistent with the principles of academic freedom, and the idea that any research on human issues could be totally objective and dispassionate was an intellectual myth. Ideas, feeling, and action constitute a kind of unity, an inseparable totality of human expression. I wrote about these issues in an article entitled "Action and Academia in the Nuclear Age" that appeared in the February 1987 issue of *Harvard Magazine*,[9] which, not surprisingly, received a range of responses from the alumni readership.

In the winter of 1979–1980 my oldest son, Daniel, then 19, came home from a weekend workshop, spread his arms wide, and declared to his startled parents, "I love you." Danny had been a somewhat competitive teenager who usually had to be right about most things. Such open expressions of loving feelings had been rare until then, and although we wondered what was going on, we were not going to look this gift horse in the mouth. He persuaded Sally and me to take the workshop, an EST spinoff that was conducted by Robert and Cynthia Hargrove. The effect of the workshop on me was to begin a process of questioning about so many of the invisible assumptions that stand in the way of loving relationships and keep us trapped in restricted world views. Danny's initiative, his taking on full strength the process of personal transformation (from which he has never turned back), helped to start me on a path of personal self-questioning and consciousness exploration that began with EST and related workshops.

Over the next years I participated in many human transformational activities, worked closely with the Esalen Institute in California in their Soviet–American exchange program, developed a halting meditation practice, and became aware of the missing development in the spiritual dimension of my nature. In September, 1987 I attended a large conference at Esalen on frontiers of health, which represented the culmination of a several-year Soviet–American health project in which I had participated that was directed by Dulce Murphy, wife of Esalen's founder Michael Murphy. Papers presented included talks by Dean Ornish on reducing coronary atherosclerosis through healthful diet and living, Robert Gale on his work at Chernobyl, and Candace Pert on the immunology of AIDs. I spoke on the nuclear war imagery that had emerged in my clinical practice with adults and children.

Stanislav Grof and his wife Christina, were in residence at Esalen at that time. Grof, a Czech-born physician and psychoanalyst, had pioneered the development of a new cartography of the mind based on his analysis of several thousand protocols of LSD experiences in patients at the Spring Grove Hospital in Maryland. These experiences revealed a deeper substrate of personality than the biographical motivational structures developed in psychoanalysis. Grof discovered that the several stages of the birth experience left a powerful imprint upon the personality and that we were also affected by what he called "transpersonal experiences," the capacity of consciousness to separate from the body and identify with any person, object or entity in the universe. Grof moved to Esalen in the 1970s to escape the restrictions on his LSD research imposed by the federal government.

With Christina, Grof developed the holotropic breathwork method, a drug-free technique for reaching the perinatal and transpersonal levels of the psyche that involves deep, rapid breathing with the eyes closed, evocative music, focal body work and mandala drawings[10] practiced in a safe, protected environment. Many thousands of individuals have attended breathwork workshops or experienced individual sessions. In addition to the profound inner healing that can occur, the breathwork method enables people to relive birth or birth-related traumata and to have powerful spiritual openings as a result of the deepening of consciousness that is associated with transpersonal experiences.

Grof offered to demonstrate the breathwork method at the end of the conference, and I eagerly, and rather anxiously, decided to participate. This experience, and many subsequent breathwork sessions, persuaded me that classical psychoanalysis was too limited a method for reaching the deeper levels of the psyche. In the first breathwork session (there were 11 of us who breathed, including two Soviet physicians who attended the conference), not much happened for about 30 minutes. But then I found myself beginning to recall images and feel powerful emotions relating to my biological mother's death, which I had not been able to access in many years of psychoanalysis, and identified deeply with my father's grief during the time thereafter, allowing me to be more forgiving of his sometimes distant ways during my early childhood. I also found myself "becoming" — not imagining exactly, but something more like being transported into another consciousness — a Russian father in the 16th century whose 4-year-old son was decapitated by Mongol hordes. The effect of this experience was to enable me to feel more empathy for the Soviet doctors at the conference and for the Russian historical experience generally. This, in turn, allowed me to be more effective in my psychopolitical work with Soviet physicians and others, as I felt more capable of seeing the Soviet–American conflict from the other side's perspective.

The creation of a nonordinary state of consciousness as occurs, for example, in hypnosis, yoga, with the judicious use of psychedelic agents, Grof breathwork, with some forms of meditation, and in shamanic journeys, I have come to feel is a vital aspect of therapeutic work that aims at achieving deep healing and personal change. Increasingly psychotherapists appear to be including some form of non-ordinary-state work in their practices. My own perinatal and transpersonal experiences in the breathwork session at Esalen affected me profoundly and led me to contact the Grofs in order to become trained and certified in the use of this method. As time permits, I continue to lead breathwork workshops and to explore how this and other non-ordinary-consciousness work relates to more traditional psychotherapeutic approaches.

Beginning in 1987, I have participated in workshops of what has come to be called the "men's movement." I have attended conferences with Robert Bly, Michael Meade, Mark Gerzon, Justin Sterling, Aaron Kipnis, Brian Muldoon, and other leaders of this movement. Contrary to the popular caricaturing of these gatherings, which would reduce them to a kind of foolish wildness, there is behind this effort a need to counter two destructive trends in American society. One is the mindless competitiveness into which men are driven by the corporate culture at the cost of their health and humanity. The other is a kind of gender homogenization in which male and female roles and sensitivities are blurred, and men are integrated into a society dominated by women's demands and values.

The men's movement in its most constructive sense is enabling men to rediscover their own identities and specific needs, their brotherhood with other men, their appropriate responsibilities as protectors at every level of society, and, finally, new ways of joining in an authentic partnership with women from a place of greater personal clarity to address the problems and grievances that beset our culture. For me personally, the contact with other men that has resulted from this participation has brought much needed companionship, closeness, and support in sometimes difficult times. I have been able to develop friendships and close bonds at a time in my life when I did not think this was possible. I wonder now how men survived in this brutalizing society without something equivalent to this movement. Perhaps in the fullest sense they haven't.

In March 1989, Stan Grof gave me a draft of a chapter on UFOs written by Keith Thompson that was soon to appear in a book edited by the Grofs on spiritual emergencies, of which a UFO encounter, in their view, might be one. I had little acquaintance with the field, but as I read Thompson's intelligent view of UFO contact as a kind of mythic crisis of transformation I kept asking myself, "But what is going on? Is it real?" A few months later, at the urging of a psychologist friend in the Grof training group, I visited Budd Hopkins, who had pioneered research in the alien abduction phenomenon. When she first told me of Hopkins' work, I had thought that the idea of humanoid beings taking people into spaceships and performing various procedures on their bodies and minds was altogether preposterous.

But the people whom Hopkins described were not, as far as I could tell, mentally disturbed, were telling stories that were highly congruent one with another, had come forth reluctantly, expressed a great deal of self-doubt, were reporting their experiences with intense distress, and provided consistent details that were not in the media. Only something that is "really" happening to people behaves like that. But if this phenomenon was in some way real, then what was its source?

This question was to occupy me for the next 4 years and resulted in the publication of a book, *Abduction: Human Encounters with Aliens,* published by Scribners in April, 1994.[11] This work was based on detailed case studies of thirteen of the more than 70 people I had interviewed before completing the manuscript who fulfilled my criteria for an abduction experiencer. These include the recollection with or without hypnosis of encountering humanoid beings, being taken forcefully into a UFO or other unfamiliar enclosure, and subjected to various intrusive procedures — all reported with affect and incredulity appropriate to what was being related and occurring in the absence of a psychiatric condition that might explain the strange account. Among these cases I had done one to nine hypnosis sessions with more than 50 individuals, for although many details of the experiences are recalled without the use of a nonordinary state of consciousness, a relaxation exercise is helpful in filling out details and in recovering the intense stressed feeling that accompanies the abduction experiences.

As I pursued this work, it became increasingly evident to me that no conventional psychiatric or even "psychosocial" explanation would be forthcoming. Whatever abductions were, they were not fantasy, dream, a new form of psychosis, or a displacement from some other kind of trauma (although, of course, the experiences themselves were often traumatic). They were what they were, i.e., in some way real, whatever that might mean. In fact, none of the now many hundreds of abduction reports in the literature has revealed behind it something else, i.e. any other condition. Abductions appear to be just what they look and sound like — a visitation of some other form of intelligence that enters people's lives in strange ways. As I first began to realize this, it seemed shocking, and, indeed, I was frequently warned not to let on, especially publicly, that I took the reports seriously and that they represented an authentic mystery. But after a time this seemed less than truthful, and I began to say in conferences, media interviews, and, of course, in the book that there seemed no logical explanation for the phenomenon other than that another intelligence was, in fact, reaching into our reality and manifesting physically as well as psychologically, even if this could not be "proven" to the satisfaction of mainstream science.

Although my work has received a great deal of interest and support, I was unprepared, even though I had been warned, for the backlash of cynicism, snide tones, and even ridicule that would greet my book, especially from some of the mainstream print media. I found myself portrayed sometimes as a kind of gullible, too-easy-to-believe Harvard professor who had taken leave of his senses. Behind this attitude lies a structure of belief, I have come to think, that regards human beings as the preeminent intelligent creatures in the cosmos, and that it is likely, if other intelligence might exist, it would behave rather like us, traveling through space by our physical laws and responding to radio signals. The notion that another intelligence might demonstrate behaviors and possess technologies and means of travel that do not follow our gravitational and other physical laws seems far-fetched to these critics, and the perception by abductees of intrusive alien beings into their lives is discounted or assumed to be some sort of hallucination, although these experiences are not at all like hallucinations. The egocentrism of this attitude, this discounting of the possible varieties of intelligence that might inhabit a multidimensional universe, seems to me to be the acme of arrogance yet achieved by our species.

As I have explored the abduction phenomenon more deeply and pondered the bitter, sometimes almost violent, resistance with which this work has been met, I have come to realize that to accept its reality means to experience that the world is altogether different than the one we, at least those of us who are the products of Western, materialist culture, assumed it was. Wars are fought not just over land and material resources but over ideas or systems of thought

— religious, political, and economic — that structure how we are to live and relate to one another and to nature itself. The UFO abductions invite a war of sorts, but it is not a military conflict fought with weapons of mass destruction. Rather, it is a struggle of fundamental world views, a "paradigm" war.

The ideological lines in this struggle are quite sharply drawn. The differences are philosophical, but the implications are pragmatic. In the materialist world view, the universe is essentially lifeless or devoid of intelligence and meaning. If intelligence is experienced as inhabiting the cosmos, this is a product of subjectivity or a projection of consciousness, which is believed to be an epiphenomenon of the human brain. If the earth is not experienced as part of a larger, perhaps delicate, intelligent system, then it becomes the potential property of any species physically and technologically powerful enough to appropriate it for its own purposes. This is, in effect, what the human species has been doing in this century, with catastrophic results for human life and the earth's living systems.

But the appreciation that the universe is filled with intelligence, and the realization that one of its infinite forms, the entities we perceive as "aliens," has found a way to enter our physical reality, possessing the capacity for interdimensional travel and the power to render us helpless, must inevitably shatter the official world view. For among the implications of this reality is the ego-destroying notion that far from being the preeminent intelligence in the universe, we are to these beings as a domestic animal is to us (although at least they do not eat us). The earth, then, far from being our oyster to devour at our pleasure, must, in this emerging world view, take its place within a cosmic design we have lost the capacity to perceive.

A practical outcome of this paradigmatic shift will be the realization that the only chance for our collective survival lies in a radical turn of direction, which, at its core, requires an expansion of the idea of who we are. In the sense that we become identified with a cosmos that is filled with intelligence and spirit, we are much larger. But insofar as we discover our lack of control and power over nature, the end of the Baconian era, we are smaller. Living in that paradox, it seems to me, can only be healthy. For then we can devote ourselves to finding a way to live in harmony with one another, other life forms on earth, and within the vast material and spiritual actuality of the universe.

In the short preface to *Abduction* I looked back on how this study related to other themes of my life's work:

> An author embarking on a venture as manifestly novel as this one must inevitably ask if some link may be found with his previous work. For me, the connection resides in the matter of identity — who we are in the deepest and broadest sense. In retrospect, this focus has been with me from the beginning, driving my clinical explorations of dreams, nightmares and adolescent suicide, my biographical researches, as well as the studies of the nuclear arms race and ethnonational conflict and, more recently, transpersonal psychology, with which I have been involved. The abduction phenomenon, I have come to realize, forces us, if we permit ourselves to take it seriously, to reexamine our perception of human identity — to look at who we are from a cosmic perspective.

This, it seems, is what my physician–activist life has been about, the discovery of identity, who I am in a personal, human, collective, and spiritual sense. That task is, at root, a psychological or inner one, and, when the suffering becomes too great, even psychiatric. Action seems called for where values are involved, when there is the experience that one's self-discoveries become generalizable and can translate into a process of transformation for others. Great joy and a good deal of suffering have, for me, been an inevitable accompaniment of the task of expanding identity. For as we break the boundaries of the self, there is both discovery and loss, richness and emptiness. Each step along the way involves an element of terror, I think, for the process involves paradox, mystery, and the unknown. In this evolution I have come to redefine faith, which always used to mean for me blind, unfounded belief. Now it means that there is a magnificent, unfolding design within the cosmos, and, if we do the work of discovering our potential place and purpose in it, that is the best we can do. This requires, however, a continuing surrender, a letting go of the illusion of control, while asking, in whatever language we have, what the divine consciousness might ask of us. This is an active process, for insofar as we experience that the evolutionary outcome is not foreordained, then we cannot escape the possibility that the next step just might depend on what each of us does.

POSTSCRIPT

Dr. John Mack continues to investigate alien abductions, focusing on how the phenomenon manifests itself in non-Western cultures. He is exploring whether the core elements of the phenonmenon are psychologically or culturally determined. "If they are neither," states Dr. Mack, "the implications of our sense of ourselves are great indeed." He is developing an outline for a book on human identity over the life span, drawing on his clinical and psychopolitical work as well as his study of human encounters with extraterrestrial beings.

REFERENCES

1. Chivian E (ed.): *Last Aid: The Medical Dimensions of Nuclear War.* San Francisco: W. H. Freedman, 1982.

2. Mack JE: *Nightmares and Human Conflict.* Boston: Little, Brown & Company, 1970. Reprinted with a revised preface, New York: Columbia University Press, 1989.
3. Mack JE: *A Prince of Our Disorder: The Life of T. E. Lawrence.* Boston: Little, Brown & Company; London: Weindenfeld and Nicholson, 1976.
4. Lawrence TE: Twenty-seven articles. In Mack JE: *A Prince of Our Disorder: The Life of T. E. Lawrence.* Boston: LIttle, Brown & Company, 1976:463–467.
5. Mack JE, Rogers RS: *The Alchemy of Survival.* Reading, MA: Addison-Wesley, 1988.
6. Cohn C: Slick 'ems, glick 'ems, Christmas trees, and cookie cutters: Nuclear language and how we learned to pat the bomb. *Bull Atomic Scientists* 1987; June:17–24.
7. Mack JE: Ideology and technology: Lessons from the Nazi doctors for the nuclear age. In Tuttman (Ed): *Psychoanalytic Group Theory and Therapy: Essays in Honor of Saul Scheidlinger.* Mew York: International University Press, 1991 45–66.
8. Mack JE: The risks of malignant professionalism in our time. Presented at the American Psychiatric Association Annual Meeting, New York, May 15, 1990.
9. Mack JE: Action and academia in the nuclear age. *Harvard Magazine* 1987;89(3):25–31.
10. Grof C, Grof S: *The Holotropic Mind.* San Francisco: Harper, 1992.
11. Mack JE: *Abduction: Human Encounters with Aliens.* New York: Charles Scribner's Sons, 1994.

INDEX